We've come a long way, sexually [...]
Healing Power of Sex was first p[...]
parts of the text, which are either factually incorrect or may give the
wrong impression.

First, the designation of homosexual men as "gays" is outdated. They
are more often referred to today as "gay men." Any list of those who
do not practice straight, heterosexual sex should include gay men, lesbians, bisexuals, and transgendered people, as well as asexual or
pansexual individuals. The mention of homosexual couples having partnerships or adopting children can now be amplified to include civil
unions and in certain states, marriage.

Any discussion of HPV (see text on page 124) must include a consideration of the new vaccine against cervical cancer for girls ages 9
through 26, a series of three which ideally should be given before the
girl becomes sexually active. The vaccine is controversial, because it is
so new and there are as yet no long-term results to report as to side
effects or adverse events. However, it does protect against four different types of HPV.

Statistics on the prevalence of prostate cancer and arthritis have
changed. Currently, eight percent of American men will develop prostate disease in their lifetime; approximately 28,660 died of it in 2008.
And over 46 million individuals in the United States suffer from
various types of arthritis.

There has been a vast rethinking of the use of replacement hormones
after menopause based on significant new evidence. (See text on
page184.) What used to be called HRT (hormone replacement therapy)
is now known as ET (estrogen therapy, for a woman without a
uterus) or EPT (estrogen-progestogen therapy for a woman with a
uterus). Where most doctors used to prescribe it routinely for women
going through "the change," it is now used far less frequently. Major
studies have shown that the risks far outweigh the benefits when we
look at incidence of breast cancer and cardiac and memory complications in later life. Most doctors now prescribe ET and EPT only to
alleviate symptoms such as hot flashes, vaginal dryness, and night
sweat, and for no more than five years. Although ET and EPT can

be helpful in staving off osteoporosis, there are other, less risky medicines for that purpose.

In the discussion about using food as part of sex play (see text on p. 258), it should be noted that no food should ever be introduced into the vaginal or anus, since it may contain bacteria and might trigger an infection.

Finally, we must acknowledge the vast power of the Internet as it relates to sexual interest and practice. How could we have imagined in 1994 that you could get any sexual experience on the Web! From online pornography to chat rooms to hooking up, the possibilities are endless.

The Healing Power of Sex

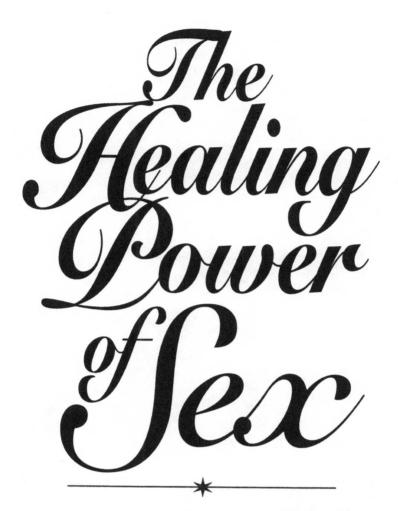

The Healing Power of Sex

JUDITH SACHS

with foreword by
DR. SANDRA R. LEIBLUM

Originially published by Prentice Hall.

Copyright © 1994 by Judith Sachs

ISBN: 978-1-5040-2891-2

Distributed in 2016 by Open Road Distribution
180 Maiden Lane
New York, NY 10038
www.openroadmedia.com

*T*o all those I have loved over the years, with passion, with conviction, with stealth, and with humor. And especially for my dearest Bruno, who helps to nourish my soul as well as my body.

Acknowledgments

To all the following, my utmost thanks for their support and information:

Barbara G. Brewer, Ph.D., University of Cincinnati

Robert Ader, Ph.D., University of Rochester School of Medicine and Dentistry

James Prescott, Ph.D., Institute for Humanistic Science

Beverly Whipple, Ph.D., R.N., College of Nursing, Rutgers University

Susan Wilson, Network for Family Life Education

Linda Crabtree, Phoenix Counsel, Inc., Ontario, Canada

Ted McIlvenna, M.Div., Ph.D., Institute for the Advanced Study of Human Sexuality

The Kinsey Institute for Sexual Research

Linda Hendrickson, Ph.D.

Gina Ogden, Ph.D.

Sandra R. Leiblum, Ph.D.

Maxine Farmer, M.S.W.

Larry Pervin, Ph.D.

Ray Rosen, Ph.D.

Enid Campbell, Ph.D.

Bob Hoyt, Ph.D.

Eric Leskowitz, Ph.D.

And to all the men and women I interviewed for this book who graciously open their hearts to tell me about the healing power of sexuality and intimacy in their lives.

$\mathcal{F}$oreword

At last! A book that enthusiastically endorses sex as not only healthy, but health promoting—sex as a positive, healing force rather than a force that promotes degradation and destruction, danger and disease.

Judith Sachs' *The Healing Power of Sex* is a welcome antidote to the negativity that characterizes much of the current sexual climate. For, in fact, sexual exchange with a loving partner can promote feelings of well-being, build self-esteem and sustain a sense of self-efficacy. When desired, it provides relief from loneliness, diminution of depression, and distraction from pain. It can, and often does, relieve tension, reduce anxiety and reinforce positive feelings about being female or male. It can lead to laughter and liberation, intimacy and engagement. It surely augers well for a sense of satisfaction in relationships—even when other things seem sour.

Sex can have even more profound effects.

We know that touch is essential to sustain and promote growth and development—both neurologically and psychologically. Infants who are touch-deprived fail to thrive. Recent research suggests that severely premature infants need tactile stimulation in order to grow normally.

Touch is also life-sustaining. Indirectly by reducing stress, sexual intimacy can promote improved immunological functioning. Stress is associated with a reduction in T-cell counts and beta-endorphin activity. Any activity that reduces stress, be it physical exercise or frolicking in bed, can enhance the body's ability to ward off disease by increasing natural killer cells and increasing endorphin production.

Research has shown that even following illness, sexual activity can promote health. For example, researchers studying men after coronary bypass surgery found that an increase in sexual frequency was related to improvement in cardiac symptoms, ability to return to work, and less type A behavior.

Unfortunately, sexual comfort and satisfaction is not all that easy to come by. Concerns about physical imperfections, fears about rejection, and conflicts about intimacy are worries for most of us.

In addition, sex-negative family messages, early life experiences, religious orthodoxy, developmental problems, sexual abuse and coercion, surgical and gynecological trauma, and disappointment in relationships all conspire to make sex problematic. Without a sense of safety and security, it is difficult to "let go" and abandon oneself to sexual pleasure.

As a sex therapist, I see individuals and couples who are disheartened and discouraged by their lack of sexual gratification: women who remain "virgin wives" because of their terror of vaginal penetration; men who feel emasculated and depressed by their inability to reliably achieve and maintain erections; and couples who have lost desire and with it the sense of closeness and intimacy they once shared.

Despite all their good intentions and heart-felt efforts, sexual fulfillment seems elusive. Guilt, anxiety, and shame accompany their sexual encounters. Sexual spontaneity and sexual self-comfort seem impossible to achieve.

It is for these reasons that *The Healing Power of Sex* is so welcome. Sachs has written a really down-to-earth, sane, and sensible book about sex. She covers everything from body image to safe sex, sex talk to treatment suggestions for common sexual difficulties. Her advice, information, and exercises provide an invaluable guide for achieving greater sexual self-acceptance and self-awareness.

Sex will not heal everything. But it can be a joyful accompaniment to life's journey. Judith Sachs has written an ebullient, enthusiastic, and eminently readable guidebook for that trip.

Sandra R. Leiblum, Ph.D.
Professor of Clinical Psychiatry
Co-Director, Center for Marital and Sexual Health
U.M.D.N.J.–Robert Wood Johnson Medical School
Piscataway, New Jersey 08854

Contents

9
How to Get More Good Sex into Your Busy Life · 163

10
How to Increase Your Sexual Energy · 193

. . . The day will come when, after harnessing the ether, the winds, the tides, gravitation, we shall harness for God the energies of love. And, on that day, for the second time in the history of the world, man will have discovered fire.

Pierre Teilhard de Chardin

Introduction

Sex.

There, I've caught your attention. You're riveted. Just the word will do it. Because the word conjures up images, memories, dreams, expectations.

Healing sex is even more intriguing. What is hurt that must be healed? What kind of remedy does sexual experience offer us? How does the miracle of a loving caress alter our lives?

Read on, and you will learn just how sex can help, heal, and hone the life skills we all depend on daily. Not only can a good sex life offer us the power to communicate and negotiate with others, it can expand our lives in ways we never dreamed possible.

Human beings crave the touch of another—without that physical connection, we can languish and die. From the moment we are picked up and held close by a mother or father, we are reassured that we are not alone on earth. And as we grow, we cherish the safe haven of two arms around us, the blessing of a kiss, the rhythm of another's breath close by, the intensity of soft or rough skin skimming ours. When we become adults, the need for intimacy includes a desire for sexual union—the ultimate bonding with another individual.

When we are born, we emerge from another person's body to enter the world and experience life. Later on, when we become sexual beings, we can enter into another person's body or receive it inside us to experience a renewal of that life.

But we do not need to put one body part inside another in order to be sexual. I'd like to encourage all manner of noninvasive sexual exploration and eroticism. Contact with hand, leg, and mouth, the experience of skin sliding against skin, the ecstatic

xix

thought that lingers in the brain and blossoms in the presence of a loved one can raise us to heights equal to that achieved in an act involving penetration.

The sexual experience joins our creative bodies and minds as nothing else can. It has a healing power that transcends medicine. A fulfilling sexual encounter is a reunion of the childlike wonder of simple things with the adult sophistication of caring for another human. And overlaid on this experience is the amazing way it raises you out of the ordinary, workaday world into a land of colors, shapes, smells, and feelings that make you bigger, stronger, better than you ever thought you were.

Sex can give you power, it can be deeply intimate, it can be casual and funny, but at its highest level, it is a form of regeneration and rebirth—the greatest healing of all. It shows us, more than any other adult activity we may participate in, the closeness that we need to share to reinforce our humanity. No matter how we value our independence and cherish our right to privacy, we have to be touched by another at some point to carry on.

If we look at our general good health as being made up of an active, responsive body, a calm mind, a well of deep emotions, and a soaring spirit—then sex is the epitome of good health. If we don't have those healthful attributes, we must cure the parts of ourselves that hold us back from gaining them.

A healing sexual experience meshes desire, comfort, and cooperation on matters as diverse as position and behavior to time, atmosphere, and setting. It touches the highs and lows of the relationship that brought it into being, even if that relationship only came into being a few hours ago. It has to be balanced—each partner must sense that he or she is both leader and follower, pursued and pursuing. And it has to end so that each person is allowed to have certain expectations for the future—even if what's wanted is to have *no* expectations.

Possibly the most important element in *healing sex* is that each person can walk away from the experience replenished with a feeling that there is something basically good and right about himself or herself.

Our upbringing and the society in which we live has taught us many false lessons about what we are supposed to do and feel when we engage in a sexual encounter. But let me make an impassioned plea for not taking those lessons to heart. We will survive longer and better when we can break out of our old expectations and forge a new meaning of sexuality that is all ours. It takes guts to do this, and practice, and a sympathettic partner or partners who are equally demanding about using their sexuality for a greater good.

Being sexual and understanding our true sexual nature can be a difficult job for some, particularly those who've been traumatized or abused physically or emotionally. What we do—and what we think we should or shouldn't do—can be so problematic, so hidden, so terrifying, that we can't even admit the truth to ourselves. We may feel bad about feeling good, or feel good and feel so guilty about it, we don't know whether we should ever feel this way again.

Dealing with our sexuality is even harder than dealing with our ideas about sex. If you don't know the difference, you will learn in the pages that follow. In the deepest recesses of your brain, heart, groin, and spirit, you will find the key to your sexuality. This key will open doors that you never knew were there. The challenge to heal yourself sexually may open up for you a part of your personality you've never explored before, with great results and wonderful benefits for the future.

What You Will Gain *from the Healing Power of Sex*

If you are unsure of yourself and your capacity for dealing with others, your sexuality will give you the power to be assertive.

If you experience chronic pain, sex will give you respite from it. You will find your pain dissolving before the pleasure that overwhelms you.

If you find it's hard to laugh in the face of career problems, money problems, personal neuroses, and children running amok, sex will restore your sense of humor.

If you feel tired and dejected, sex will give you a lift.

Whether or not you are an orgasmic phenomenon, you will find that you are more at home in your *body* when you rely on your sexuality to heal you. You will learn how your *mind* creates a sensory palace of wonders to explore. You will find untapped *emotions* and become expert at sharing them with a partner. And you may actually discover your ineffable *spirit*. So much appears to be possible sex-

sex out of the bedroom and bring it into your everyday life. When you can translate the warmth, the consideration, the excitement, the passion and the energy you generate in a sexual setting to any other situation, you can effectively become a healthier person.

Sex and health have been rudely split apart in the past decade, due to the terrifying spread of a variety of sexually transmitted diseases, including human immunodeficiency virus (HIV) disease. For this reason, the emphasis in many circles is on protecting yourself from your partner when you slip between the sheets. This book, however, shows you how to tap the healing power of your sexuality and sow the seeds of good sexual health among your lovers, colleagues, and friends and in the world in general. When you approach sex from the perspective of all the good it can do, you immediately reap the benefits.

This book pulls no punches. It is a guide for those brave enough to explore a world that they may have ignored or denigrated in the past. Talking about your sexuality is really the best means of learning what you want, and there are several chapters devoted to being verbally explicit so that you can bring out your feelings, fears, and joys with your partner.

Many of us were wounded by the old restrictions and superstitions handed down by earlier generations who were terrified of sex. In healing the past, we can heal the future. Because we can leave our own children a positive legacy, they will be able to do the same for their children. We owe a debt to them to provide them with a sane, joyful perspective on their sexuality. The chapter on talking to your children may be a difficult one for many to read and *use*, but it's essential.

Finally, to make the best use of this book, you must take it out of the realm of the strictly sexual and let it touch all aspects of your life. The healing power of sex—which gives us freedom, warmth, compassion, a sense of self, an ability to merge with another—all these wonderful qualities can be incorporated into everything else we do.

Several years ago, after I wrote a book about menopause and midlife, I began teaching workshops to men and women who were going through significant life changes. I found that the most turbulent feelings, either expressed or denied, centered on their sexuality. As I've explored this territory more fully in my workshops and in my personal life, I have discovered the urgent need for information, reassurance, and comfort—that is the purpose of this book. But it is also an invitation to all of you, no matter your age or life situation, to start to explore within and without and delve into darker corners of your sexuality. There, you may be surprised to find a great deal of illuminating light.

You will gain many benefits from this journey. You will learn that healing sexuality may be hard won; that it doesn't all happen in bed or in the back seat of a car; that you have to talk about it even if it's embarrassing; that sexual health has many factors—physical, mental, emotional, social, and spiritual; that just because something worked before doesn't mean you shouldn't keep experimenting and playing around. *Playing around*, sometimes jokingly, sometimes seriously, but always with joy and excitement, is what sex is all about. Good play leads to good health.

The most influential sexual organ in the body is the mind. When we believe we are attractive, first to ourselves and then to others, we have the power to change the way we approach life. We can mold and shape what we want to do when we leave the bedroom because we've treated ourselves and another well. We have the mandate to experience life—not just pure sensation and physical pleasure (which are awfully nice as far as they go, but there's a lot farther we can take them if we're willing to).

Why wait? It's all yours now, if you will simply agree to change your mind. In changing your mind, you can bind up the old wounds of your past and grow a new sexual skin. The emergence from old expectations is like that great moment after your first kiss. Passionate kissing looked strange, even disgusting, to you when you were a kid; then, as you started to experiment with your own arm or the pillow or the mirror to see what it might feel like, it seemed impossible to get any pleasure from this activity.

But one day, it all changes. You feel deeply for another, you are held and hold on for dear life in an embrace, and suddenly, you discover the key to your sexuality. With this amazing key—this healing power—you can open the doors of your mind, heart, and soul.

1

Why Sex Is Good for You

$\mathcal{P}$eel back the skin of almost any adult relationship and you will find a throbbing core of sexuality. You may deny this on first reflection, but give me a minute. Don't look at the surface, but see what's really going on as two physical and emotional beings get in touch with each other. Go through a list of people you know in your head and consider the possibilities. The dynamic boss, always ready with a new idea or strategy; the kind schoolteacher, nurturing and always available; the neighbor who teaches aerobics, fairly pulsing with dynamism as she walks down the street.

What gives them their spark? Partly, it's creativity, and an ability to reach out to others. But it's also an energy, an appetite for life.

These people exude an aura of life-affirming spirit that makes them look good, feel good, and appear in harmony with those around them. They are excited about what they do in the world, and this excitement pervades every aspect of what they see, touch, feel, and do. Whether they are lying in bed with their lover or are standing up at a town council meeting expressing an opinion, they are filled with physical, mental, and emotional drive. They attract—perhaps even entice or seduce—others to their way of thinking because they have that certain something. They are permeated with a glow of good health that works for them and for everyone who comes into contact with them.

We desire the touch of others from our first moments on earth; without touch, we would never have the will to take our first steps, speak our first words, or join in with the rest of humanity to make our mark on the world. The sexual act is just one way that we touch, but the part of our personality that makes us sexual beings is working constantly. And it is this amazing, mysterious, powerful element that cleanses our body, sharpens our wits, warms our soul—*total sexuality*—that we will explore in this book.

2

$\mathcal{D}$o You Have What It Takes to Be Sexually Healthy?

If you want to be sexually healthy, you must first

- be comfortable with your chosen gender and sex role and accept yourself without shame, guilt, or fear.

- be able to maintain good relationships with both sexes, regardless of whether they are platonic or intimate.

- have the ability to become aroused—if you choose to be—when given any form of erotic stimulation—tactile, aural, visual, and so on.

- have the ability to make mature judgments on your sexual behavior and choices that coincide with your personal values and beliefs.

- be free of organic disorders and diseases that may interfere with your sexual or reproductive capacity.

- be conscientious about protecting yourself and your partners from any disease transmission.

It is quite a responsibility, then, to be sexually healthy. You must be sound of body and mind, and even be mature. It's much easier to get into good cardiovascular shape or take care of your bones— no one ever questions your moral values when you sign up for a fitness program.

I think one of the reasons it's hard to put a finger on the exact nature of sexual health is that we have no guidelines to govern it. Despite the fact that we condone and sometimes watch NC-rated movies, wear highly suggestive clothing, and feel comfortable discussing who slept with whom at the office, the real information about our sexuality is still kept in the dark. If we only knew what everybody else was doing in bed or what their fantasies were like, we wouldn't feel so strange, awkward, and out of line. Are we repressed? Are we perverted? Do we want sex too much or too little? There's no barometer.

We *know* that our cholesterol level should hover around 200 and that we should engage in some form of daily physical exercise.

We've been *told* that we can avoid cancer if we do self-exams and have mammograms and prostate checks on a regular basis. It is drummed into us from childhood that we can keep our teeth and gums healthy by flossing and brushing twice daily. But no one ever tells us what to do about sexual health, and they don't even divulge what other people are doing.

What are we going to do if nobody hands us a list of the rules? We have to make them up as we go along. And that's a pretty awesome prospect for many. How do I reassure myself that I'm okay sexually? I look in the mirror and I'm not sure how desirable this body is. I sit across a table from a new prospective partner and I'm so tongue-tied by the thought of starting a relationship that I lose all the words in my vocabulary. Suppose my desires aren't "normal"? Suppose they don't coincide with fantasies my new partner is too embarrassed to confide to me? Unfortunately, the fact that we keep our sexuality closed up most of the time gives us plenty of opportunity for ruminating about our imperfect bodies, techniques, appeal, what have you.

We cannot find out about our sexuality by comparing ourselves to our friends, relations and movie stars. If we're looking to be—or to sleep with—"a perfect 10," we're doomed. Because nobody, except in fantasy, is perfect.

What Makes Sex Sexy?

There's so much going on at once! The experience of wanting and pursuing sexual intimacy is fascinatingly complex. Sex is a multilayered, multileveled experience that takes place simultaneously on biological, psychological, emotional, and social planes.

Biology

The process starts in the *limbic system*, a primitive and instinctive part of the brain. Among other functions, it serves as the pleasure center of the body, and it drives us to search out experiences that will enhance the way we feel about ourselves. Our pleasure center demands that we remain warm, fed, and safe from harm and that we satisfy the overwhelming need all of us have to link up physically and emotionally with another.

The higher-echelon brain functions that afford us sophisticated decision-making skills are located in the *cerebral cortex*. It is in this region of the brain that we decide on partners, times, and places for sexual encounters. The wondrous circuitry of the body allows brain stimulation to trigger hormonal responses in our genitals and neurotransmitter and neuropeptide responses in our nervous systems.

Personality

The way we feel about ourselves governs the way we perceive our attractiveness to others. Our fears, hopes, dreams, stresses, mental state, and other factors allow us to go toward or retreat from a potential lover.

Shy people may have torrential sexual feelings that can emerge only when they truly trust their partner. Those who tend to be gregarious in everyday life may turn into quiet, receptive sexual partners. You may find your personality changing in bed—some of your problems dissipating, others magnifying. But if you are able to stop relying on your image of what makes you interesting or appealing, you get to break the chains that may hold you back from freer expression of the way you feel. The bedroom is one place where you can play with your personality and try on lots of new hats. They may not all fit, but your willingness to explore will give you a wider perception of the person you are.

Life Experience

If we've had a childhood trauma such as incest or abuse, if we are physically, mentally, or emotionally challenged or disabled, if we've had an accident or illness or are in chronic pain, if we are succumbing to the aging process, these things will play a large part in our sexual options.

Your early sexual years may be a big determinant of how you mature sexually. If you had a wide variety of sexual experience in your teens and twenties, you may have trouble adjusting to a monogamous life-style later on. If you got married right out of high school and divorced in your forties or fifties, you may feel overwhelmed with the hassles of dealing with the singles' marketplace—

vastly complicated these days by the dangers of sexually transmitted disease. You can never forget your past or the positive and negative sexual choices you made—but that's a good thing. When you allow these choices to inform your future, you grow immeasurably as a sexual being. There is always room to make yourself sexually healthier than you have been if you keep your mind and heart open.

Social Factors

Our family background, our moral and religious beliefs, our conviction and comfort about our sexual preferences and orientation, the relationships that we choose, and the overall wash of our response to society's expectations for us will shape and define our behavior—at least for part of our lives.

The Victorians covered sex with heavy drapery, but their bizarre practices are legend. The commune-dwellers of the 1960s cried "Free Love!" and wailed bitterly twenty years later when the first cases of HIV infection were diagnosed. Those who dare to reconfigure the notion of sexuality always learn that this precious gift cannot be taken for granted.

But the curious and wonderful thing about society's self-correction is that we are able to prove, over and over, that no one group has the right idea or the right to say they have a right idea. And although we're all so terribly influenced by what our bunch, our clan, or our neighbors are doing, there's no way we can function in a sexually healthy manner when we rely solely on the rules of the group. We have to be brave enough to dance around the borders of society's expectations.

How to Say Yes to Life with Healthy Sex

Life-affirming sex with a compassionate partner is good for you. It can take the place of medicine, and its effects can be long-lasting. It can quell such demons as loneliness, anxiety, tension, timidity, depression, touch deprivation, psychological trauma, and alienation. It can actually relieve chronic pain, stiffness, body ache, and insomnia and alleviate certain skin disorders. It can restore you to yourself.

If you perceive sex as beneficial, it can enhance your feeling and body state of comfort, excitement, closeness, and bonding. If you've been abused or conditioned to react with fear or anger to a sexual encounter, then sex won't be good until you have the right partner and circumstance to change the way you see yourself in this type of situation.

There are biochemical, neurological, and electrical changes that go on in the body throughout arousal, plateau, orgasm, and resolution (Masters and Johnson's designated four stages of sexual experience). If you feel cherished and wanted, if you are transported by ecstatic waves of well-being, if you have the physical release of orgasm, you can in fact feel more fulfilled and willing to take on the challenges of the day. There are numerous documented cases of the healing power of touch. The interesting part about "laying-on-of-hands," which has been an acknowledged method of curing illness for centuries, is that touch alone can't do it.

Controlled experiments have shown that when a healer puts his or her hands on a patient, the energy can't get through unless there's warm, compassionate feeling passing from hand to body and back again. The concern of the healer, the relationship of the two people, the power of determination that must be present has a lot to do with the effect.

In a workshop I taught at a holistic center a couple of years ago, I was privileged to be a part of a group ritual healing. The leader explained to the 140 women present that those who had some ailment or injury they wanted the group to work on should come up and lie on the mats she had placed around the room. The rest of us could either move around the room and chant a healing song or be with the women on the mats. It didn't matter that we had no idea what we were doing. We were healers because we wanted to be.

I knelt by the side of a woman in her early thirties and gingerly touched her shoulder. There were at least six others laying hands on her feet, her thighs, her head, her belly. We encased her in our energy, and the sounds of the women keening around us generated a vibration I've never felt before. Some wonderful energy coursed through all of us. The woman on the mat started shaking, and I held my ground, feeling a new force in my hands that didn't come from me. She started crying, and her body shook with power. She appeared to enter an orgiastic state, where she forgot her pain and allowed the intimate care given by the group to heal her. The touch we had applied took over—we had no intention any more, no will to make her stronger. It just happened.

I was humbled by this extraordinary event. At the end of the hour and a half, the intensity of feeling in the room was palpable. The 140 of us had created something together, which had permitted a second stage of work to begin where we no longer had to create but instead became part of the creation. The healed woman I had touched said to us afterward, "I couldn't tell where you began and I left off. The energy you poured out mixed with mine, and at first that hurt a lot. But soon it changed, and I was carried on waves of love from all of you."

I was sure that the energy source we tapped into in that room was sexual as well as healing. The laying-on-of-hands that happens between two people creates its own special force field; imagine the power of the laying-on-of-hands of 140. The energy we supplied gave birth to a generative power that no one can measure by scientific parameters. Did her tumor dissolve? Was she healed? I will never know. But I do know that everyone who participated in this incredible experience formed an intimate bond with one another. They left their own concerns to get inside another body, another life, and fill it with strength and love.

As we will see in following chapters, people suffering from chronic pain can tap into this type of sexual power. Pain thresholds are elevated during sex, which acts as a potent anesthetic when necessary. Sleep patterns can be altered and improved. Hormonal and neurotransmitter secretion, integral to the sexual act, can have ramifications for the health of other body systems.

Experience the Power of Sexual Union

Even if you don't love your partner, you may experience a lessening of depression and anxiety if you are mentally and physically rewarded by being sexual with this person. Why does the healing work? Because when we are lifted out of our daily concerns and give ourselves over to the enormous power that is generated in a sexual union, we can let go of our pain, wherever we hold it. We gain perspective and a new way of seeing ourselves—the free, uninhibited joy of coming is a mental as well as a physical tonic.

Could we be healthier if we had more *good*, affectionate, caring sex? Could we stay well for decades if we always had access to intimate touch? My answer is yes. The feeling state we enter when we're sexually awake and aware is sufficient to alleviate a variety of ills, both physical and emotional. The relative importance of sexual well-being in our lives depends entirely on our attitude. If you think that eating an apple a day will keep you well, that may do just as much for you as an orgasm a day will do for me.

Horny Hamsters Stay Well

The evidence from lower forms of life in the laboratory is startling and very persuasive. Golden hamsters allowed to copulate freely remained healthy even after being injected with cancer-causing drugs, whereas their celibate compatriots sickened and died from the same injections. Laboratory animals with higher androgens (the male sex hormone that is responsible for our libido) not only had increased sex drives but also increased the number of T-cells (white blood cells of the immune system that help to fight off disease before it can take hold).[*]

It will be interesting to see, in the coming years, as science becomes more sophisticated and is better able to tease out the various elements in our minds and bodies and in society at large, what conclusions may be drawn about human sexuality and good health.

---

[*]"Sexual Behavior Suppresses the Primary Antibody Response in the Golden Hamster," Ostrowski, N.L. and Kress, D.W., *Brain, Behavior and Immunity* 3, 61–71 (1989).

How Sex, Sexual Behavior, and Sexuality Promote Good Health

Sex is one of the instinctive drives we have to survive and remain comfortable, just like thirst, hunger, and avoiding pain.

Sexual behavior is the type of participation we have with ourselves or others involving the genitals and other erogenous zones.

Sexuality includes the first two elements as well as the emotional, social, and spiritual components—the complex personalities, relationships, and feelings involved that draw us together on a human level.

The reason that we can be healthier if we maintain a healthy sex life is that this process doesn't only take place when we're making love—it spills over into our daily work and home life. Everything that promotes an expanded sense of our sexuality also promotes our good health in general—taking our physical needs seriously, being creative, feeling all our emotions deeply and fully, healing original family issues, experiencing something in life greater than the limited self, establishing a network of friends and acquaintances, communicating our needs and wishes, and finally, gaining a spiritual sense of why we're here on earth in the first place.

The Four Elements of Sexual Power

Being sexually healthy means that you know how to use the four elements of sexual power:

1. You have a well-developed sense of self.

2. You are able to establish and maintain good relationships.

3. You have an internal and external obligation to your partner to keep both of you physically and emotionally well. This means that you not only practice safer sex (see Chapter Five), but you also have a respect and reverence for your partner's feelings.

Finally, to be really sexually healthy,

4. You must exude a positive energy that is catching—others see you as attractive because you radiate this ecstasy for life that goes beyond what you look or sound like or how much money

you have or whether you're gay, straight, bi, married, single, or still considering your options.

A Positive Self-image and Healthy Sex Go Together

If you don't like yourself, how can you offer your mind, heart, and soul to another? You're on shaky ground when you begin to trust enough to make the decision to sleep with another person, or even to take him or her in your arms. Suppose they don't like the way you move or smell? Suppose they want to do something you find repellent or frightening?

All this stuff to consider, and that's just at the opening of the show. Suppose it goes on past a few weeks or months and you fall in love, but the other person doesn't? How will you cope with it; what will you do for yourself to make it all right again?

When we are children, the seeds are sown for the way we will feel about ourselves for years, perhaps for the rest of our lives. If our parents instill in us a good sense of ourselves, we can take it from there and nurture that feeling as we grow more independent and are able to see how effective we can be in the world.

If, on the other hand, we are abused or denigrated as children, if we're made to feel that we have to apologize just for being here, it takes a great deal to work our way out of that pit. Layers upon layers of meaning and intention and denial go into our burgeoning self-esteem or lack of it.

Some children are more resilient than others; some can't take the heat. Rejection is a powerful tool in the hand of a parent, and it may be replayed over and over as we grow. Many men interviewed for this book told me that the worst moment they could recall was the first time they tried to kiss a companion and were rebuffed. "The fact that I'd screwed up, that she didn't want me, that I was probably repulsive to her so how could I have suggested it, made me really cringe," confessed Jack, a concert pianist who had no doubts about his own worth in other parts of his life. "I questioned my ability to do this thing, to ever be able to please another person."

Everyone's perception of his or her ability to go out to others is different, and our needs and desires to be sexual often change with our stage of life. Some individuals are content to walk their own path, but most of us look to friends, relatives, or what we read in the newspapers to see what's "normal." And then we start to fabricate, based on what we think is expected of us sexually. There are undoubtedly sensitive people masked as macho and brave souls masquerading as tender shoots. People rarely tell the truth about their sexuality—even to themselves.

What are you as a sexual being? How did you come to this style of behavior? Were you conscious of a time when you changed yourself to conform to what your family or the media or some fantasy image dictated? If your self-esteem is shaky, there is no way that you can express yourself sexually in a free and open manner, without regard to society's expectations. When the stuff you think you're supposed to want becomes all mixed up with your personal inclinations, it's difficult to sort out what you really wanted in the first place.

Part of the problem is the difference between what we perceive as "normality" and "perfection" in terms of our sexual behavior.

- Do I do what everyone else does?
- Do I do it as much or as rarely?
- Do I enjoy it as much as everyone else?
- Is there something wrong with me if I don't enjoy it?
- Why doesn't it end up as fabulous as I expected it would?
- How could I change my sex life to make it better, richer, more connected to the rest of what I do every day?

The good feelings you have about yourself are not solely sexual, of course, but if you acknowledge your sexuality as an integral part of your personality, you will start to see how it touches on everything else. Your effectiveness as a speaker, your creativity at your job, your willingness to cajole a cranky child into play is all built around your sense of well-being. To put your feelings about yourself in perspective and to see how healthy you might be sexually, let's start with a definition of good health in general.

What Is Good Health?

In a recent study at the Center for Biomedical Ethics at Stanford University, individuals were asked to evaluate what it was that made them consider themselves "healthy." Men and women were uniformly together on the fact that good health was a global feeling—it encompassed physical, mental, emotional, spiritual and social elements. What gave them deep satisfaction was the interplay between health, a sense of self, body, and gender.

The body comes first. We have to nourish it, move it in space, and swaddle it in sufficient clothing for the climate. We have to decorate it and preen as our tribal ancestors did. And we need another's eyes to offer appreciation and true satisfaction in the way we are as individuals. What keeps the tribe alive is the vibrancy and juice we all supply with our passions and self-interests. Once we've satisfied ourselves, we can satisfy another and the group as a whole.

The big factors for all the respondents in this study were friends and family, food, rest, and exercise. The people in this survey also said that health was a fluctuating state—it could be changed by outer or inner forces.

One woman said, "Health is being balanced in the things you do." Finally, some added that loving and being loved was a component of good health. The elements of feeling and being healthy extend way beyond the individual.

What Is Good Sex?

I wholeheartedly agree with that woman—everything in the universe demands balance. If we are out of sync with ourselves or those around us, we feel ineffective, fatigued, hopeless, lacking in creative energy. When we achieve a good mix of leading and following, thoughtfulness and spontaneity, lightness and intensity, we feel better about ourselves and the world around us.

Sex is usually described in hot terms, as fire, burning, smoldering, igniting. But if we allowed ourselves to be consumed by this hot element, we'd be goners. There must be a cooling edge to our passion to balance it. Water, the most predominant element in our body structure, represents the other side of our emotional responsiveness. It quenches fire, but it can also temper our quick energies and give us peace. Water can be a languid pool, but is often a rushing stream, a torpid whirlpool, or an ever-changing sea. Many people talk about their orgasms—hot as they may be—as similar to the ocean waves.

There is a third element in good, balanced sex, and that is more difficult to define. It is the essence, or ether, the spirit that comes from the wavelike passion. Those who have achieved a very high level of sex talk about a meeting of souls, a purity and unity in their connection with a lover. There are actual methods used (see Chapter Thirteen) that will channel the heated business of sex into a spiritual bond that goes beyond words, touch or feelings.

Fire	*Water*	*Spirit*
Passion	*Temperance*	*Bonding*

These three elements that we all carry within us comprise the best of our sexuality. To be more concrete about this, we can say that *good sex is an extension of good health*:

- Our fire element makes us take responsibility for the most crucial part of human relationships, that is, how deeply we wish to align ourselves—even to the point of creating new life—with another individual.

- Our water element balances our need for privacy with our need to reach out to others.

- It also manifests hidden emotions with very substantial actions and sensual responses like touching, smelling, seeing, hearing, and tasting.

- Our spirit element makes us aware that we are not alone in this journey through the decades. Sexuality is a wake-up call to life; it brings home to us most clearly the zing and pizzazz of years well lived.

Rob, a sixty-two-year-old New England minister interviewed for this book, said, "Sex isn't episodic; it flows out of you or it doesn't. People can function sexually if that's all they're capable of, but those who are deeply committed to their sexuality are sexual all the time. If you're plugged into it," he said, "you use it in the same way you use any other skill you've mastered in life."

Good sex should allow us to make our own decisions in conjunction with a partner—how much we want to give or receive, how routine or spontaneous we are, how joyfully we play with one another, how many and what kind of risks we choose to take.

It should improve the quality of our life (in fact, if we look at the increasing evidence for active sexuality in extreme old age in Chapter Eight, we may decide it also increases the quantity of life). Being healthy, as we've seen, is a harmonious state of balance where mind, body, and spirit feel as if they're functioning on all cylinders. Then the feeling we have about ourselves when we're involved in a sexual relationship that eases pain, relieves physical and emotional tension, satisfies our soul, and gives us that "glow" can be truly symphonic.

What Is Unhealthy Sex?

Sex that is nonconsensual is unhealthy. Any sexual act that injures, degrades or humiliates another individual is unhealthy. Any sexual act that involves an adult coercing a minor child to perform with or for him or her is unhealthy.

But hugging and touching a child is wonderful—too many adults avoid embracing children because they fear their own sexuality and think that anything physical may be regarded as erotic. Not so. It can be extremely unhealthy to avoid any contact with others just because you think it may be construed in a sexual manner.

In this day of overabundant lawsuits, we are all being careful. Employees watch their eyes and mouths in the workplace. Soldiers and sailors are being reminded that an inappropriate innuendo can start a war. Doctors are sensitive to their patients' desire for a nurse to be present when they're being examined. That's probably not a bad thing, because there has in fact been so much revolting misuse of sexuality in the past. It is unhealthy sexual behavior to treat another person like a collection of body parts to be ogled, commented on, and fondled. The recent clamp-down on harassment in the workplace is a correct response to unthoughtful behavior gone haywire.

But where do you cross the line between sexual aggressiveness and good old affectionate appreciation? The line is very fine, and must be drawn again and again between consenting individuals. When you learn to say what you want and don't want, you are well on your way to sexual health.

*C*hoosing Your Approach to Sexual Health

There is no one path, because all paths are right if you and your partner are feeling good and giving each other what you want. The individuals interviewed for this book, and those who have participated in studies on sexuality since the days of Kinsey, report many feelings of commonality. At the same time, each is unique in his or her desires and practices, and in the way they perceive sexuality changing for them across the lifespan.

We will meet many wonderful people in the chapters that follow, men and women who have allowed me a very intimate glimpse of their sexual past and present, and none of them had the same approach to their sexual good health. For now, let's look at four possible paths:

- Mark equates good sex with good caring. He had a wonderful marriage that ended in his wife's death from cancer, but the women he meets now don't have the sense of sharing and play that he requires in a mate. He says that he could not love a person physically without feeling a deep spiritual bond.

- Alice is not afraid of the hotter elements of her sexuality, and she welcomes experiences that many of us would shun. She is able to separate her ideas about "love" and "sex." Alice, though very happily married for the last twenty years, has an intimate relationship with another man she feels is her "body-mate." Alice is deeply involved in the richness of her sexuality.

- Angela has been on the dark side and come across. She was molested by her father and gang-raped the summer she graduated elementary school, but she was determined not to be crushed. As an adult, therapy and what she terms "the basic natural force of sex in my life" affected a cure for her. She credits her ability to feel again to a strong mental and emotional core, and the desire to heal her past and her sexuality together.

- Hannah chose a different path from the one condoned by society. Married twice to men she never really connected with, she is currently in a healthy long-term relationship with a woman, Hannah doesn't like the classification of "lesbian." Rather, she is someone who is open enough to conceive of a larger picture of her own sexuality and can let it nourish the rest of her life.

How did these individuals come to their particular brand of sexuality? How did you? Has it always been there, or did it grow with your personality, your body, your spirit?

If you are able to expand your view of yourself as a sexual being, someone who doesn't just "have sex" but "is sexual," you will simultaneously develop a greater ability to enjoy life. Sex is good for you because it reinforces everything else you are and you do. If you eat a well-balanced diet, exercise daily, take some private time to meditate or simply be by yourself, you have gifted yourself with a healthy life-style.

These stepping stones of good health lead along the pathway to a more sophisticated type of self-help—that is, awareness of your instincts, drives and motives, likes and dislikes, and sense of your own self-worth. When you like yourself, you are able to move onto the next stage, where you get involved with others you like and who appreciate you. A healthy approach to your relationships then develops whereby you can accept others for what they have to give you without attempting to mold them into some unrealistic image you might have of them.

If you have all of this, consider what this does to your most intimate bondings. You desire a closeness—body and soul—and your desire matches your partner's. By taking care of your physical, mental, and emotional health, you have learned to generate warmth and accept the healing touch of those who care about you.

Think of your sexuality as a great river—the flowing energy from one tributary meets and matches that of another. Until finally, the waters come together and no one can tell where one started and another ended. They are one. Your sexual health becomes a mirror of your general good health and vice versa.

But first you have to spend time to get to know yourself sexually, and this isn't something most of us have a lot of practice doing. So let's begin with a step-by-step guide that will offer you insight into your good health and your sexuality. Celebrate the amazing colors and enjoy the ride.

How
Sex Works:

The Mind–Body
Connection

*I*n 1970, when I was twenty-three, I stopped menstruating. I wasn't a marathon runner or a ballet dancer, nor had I experienced any particular trauma that might have shocked my system into stony recalcitrance. Then followed eight years of incredible machinations on the part of the medical establishment I consulted to get me back on my hormonal track again. There was talk of infertility, of cancer, of emotional imbalance. The pharmacological and surgical monkeyshines I subjected myself to in the name of science did no particular harm, and may have done some good. But no medical professional I consulted seemed to have a clue as to what had gone wrong in my mysterious endocrinological kingdom.

In 1978, I met the man I eventually married. I was wary at first, because I didn't really believe that we could be as glued together as we clearly were. Then I was incredibly, totally sexually overwhelmed. The abundance of sex between us was delightful, funny, warm, stimulating, powerful. Then, I was in love, feeling that this person and I had a kind of linkage that wasn't purely social or purely physical but constantly evolving. We appeared to be two individuals with one drive for life that eventually metamorphosed into individual drives with a unified existence.

From the first month of our sexual involvement, my periods were regular and uneventful, and I celebrated each one (sometimes quietly, sometimes with a smug little dance), until we decided to get pregnant in 1984. We conceived the first month we tried and our daughter was born without complications on New Year's Eve.

What happened inside me? Was all this *angst* I suffered around the issue of my ovaries, glands, and hormones due to some wacky set of biochemical errors, was it all in my mind, or was there a significant alteration in my inner wiring when my emotional life took charge of my physical dysfunction?

This is not a question I can answer definitively, but I will make a stab, given the new body of scientific evidence that attempts to show how body and mind are interconnected.

The Great Circle of Sexuality: Mind, Body, and Life Force

To make this as simple as possible, let us think about the impetus toward sexuality in our lives as a driver getting in a car filled with gasoline to drive to the shore. The driver is the *mind*, the car is the *body*, and the gas is the *life force* that spurs the system to action. The car would go nowhere if the driver didn't make the decision to take the trip, didn't fill up the tank, and didn't start up the engine. But, on the other hand, the driver would be stuck in town if he didn't have a car, if it wasn't running, or if he didn't have gas money. The elements are interdependent, just as mind, body, and spirit are in the sexual act.

Cars run (so I've been told) not because of any one factor but because many different systems work in harmony—the fuel system, the cooling system, the hydraulic brake system, the steering, suspension, shock absorbers, the battery, the ignition, the valves, pistons, crankshaft, radiator, windshield wipers—I could go on! Together they are all responsible for the final result: a car tooling down the road.

The body, mind, and spirit or life force also depend on one another. If the driver (the mind) didn't have the volition or interest or social awareness of sex, he'd never fill the car up with gasoline. The gas (the life force) is the spark of something that gets us going sexually, whether that something is desire or arousal, or maybe the very basic pull toward survival of the species that moves us to procreate. The driver also has at his command enhancers of the sexual experience (the mind's ability to perceive the five senses) to make him acutely present in the moment, and his libido, that part of the personality that drives us to be sexually active.

There are external forces, too. If you lived in a tribal society where women were expected to take many sexual partners, you would never have heard the word "slut," because that concept wouldn't be in the language of your tribe. If you lived in a monastery where celibacy was the expectation and the rule, you would be ostracized if you brought home a *Playboy* magazine. The social group of which you are a member determines to a great extent where you will go on your particular car trip.

Now what happens after you fill your tank with gas? You can look at the gross anatomy and see that the genital organs are there like all those pipes and wires under the hood, ready to be active. But the penis would never become erect, the vagina would never become richly lubricated, nor would other exciting events occur afterward unless a variety of biochemical, electrical, cognitive and emotional changes happened first. Let us go back to the brain, the overriding organ that starts the system going.

Sex, the Brain, and the Central Nervous System

Deep within the brain is the *limbic system*. This system, which houses a very important gland called the *hypothalamus*, controls temperature, blood pressure, blood sugar, and our internal clock. It is also the repository of emotional reactions, specifically sex and aggression (the "fight-or-flight" response). Our pleasure and pain centers reside in the limbic system.

The *neocortex*, or the top layer of the brain (where the right and left hemispheres divide), also plays a crucial role in your sexuality. The right brain is nonverbal, just like your limbic system; the left is responsible for language and organization. The two hemispheres are held together by the *corpus callosum*, a bundle of nerve fibers. Some sexologists feel that we can bridge this gap and unite the two sides of the brain temporarily during the orgasmic state where we experience a transcendental rapture that rises above the mere physical sensation of release.

The average brain is a factory staffed by about 100 billion cells called neurons that are constantly relaying information back and forth to one another. Electrical impulses travel along the branchlike extensions of the nerve cell to its nucleus, and this causes a release of chemicals called *neurotransmitters*. These nerve stimulants act as messengers between nerve synapses. That rush of delight—the tingle in the penis and the wetness in the vagina—that's triggered when your lover whispers something delicious in your ear—is caused by neurotransmitter release.

The brain could not communicate with the rest of the body, and our car would never move, were it not for the *nervous system*. Neurotransmitters carry their messages beyond the brain down the spinal cord and out to every part of the body. When you anticipate the moment when your lover walks in the door after you've had an argument, your brain tells your adrenal glands to produce the neurotransmitters adrenalin and norepinephrine. If you're under a lot of stress—going through a difficult divorce or covering up an extramarital affair, for example—the quantity of neurotransmitters you produce can actually depress your immune system, making you more prone to illness.

Another set of brain regulators, the *neuropeptides*, include the *endorphins*, the natural opiates produced by the brain during strenuous physical activity or sexual intercourse, or when we experience pain. Endorphins block pain, but we experience their effect as that well-being and euphoria that can overcome the distractions, frustrations and physical twinges we may experience. Even if you're coupled with your lover on a prickly bed of pine needles with a rock for your pillow, the endorphins you produce during orgiastic ecstasy block out any discomfort.

There's a close link between pleasure and pain. The Marquis de Sade explored this phenomenon thoroughly in his writings. He truly believed that the deepest forms of sexual ecstasy were attained through excruciating pain—up to and including torture and death. De Sade was a disturbed individual, but even those of us who can make appropriate distinctions between pain and pleasure often find the experiences melding during sex. It's possible to be bitten or scratched during the act of love and derive rapturous pleasure from the pangs of pain. We are transported, carried away by the intensity of the moment, and our boundaries blur.

A baby's first exposure to the world often dictates how he or she will react to sensory stimulation later. Any form of sensory deprivation at birth, like not being able to get enough air because the umbilical cord is wrapped around the neck, can damage the sensory receptors and prevent the normal development of that part of the brain that tells us a touch is desirable. A baby who is slapped more than he's hugged will come to regard the hostile touch as appropriate. His brain will release endorphins when his body is abused, and in later life, this may result in violent behavior. The baby who is constantly held and rocked, on the other hand, will always cherish the softness and activity of good touch—this is the child who will probably grow up to be a wonderful lover.

Sex and the Endocrine System

The hypothalamus in the brain triggers a chain reaction of hormonal stimulation. A *hormone* (which in Greek means to "stimulate or excite") is another type of chemical messenger that travels from gland to gland, priming its target gland like a pump and getting it ready for action.

The hypothalamus communicates with the pituitary, which in turn delivers hormonal messages to the sexual organs. And these organs produce hormones that direct the sexuality show. Men produce testosterone in their testes; women produce estrogen and progesterone in their ovaries. But the adrenal glands allow us to cross-reference our gonadal hormones: Women also produce some testosterone, which enhances libido, and men produce some estrogen.

When our hormones start to rage in adolescence, we are overcome by every whiff of sex that comes our way. As testosterone levels rise in boys, they can think about virtually nothing but the next erection—which for most arrives at the most unexpected moments, and frequently. Girls may be moody and distracted, but they too feel the pull of their hormonal tides. A girl's libido is complicated by society's expectations that she keep those feelings under wraps, but there's no dictating to estrogen and the androgens—she is clearly ready and willing for experimentation at this time.

Sex and the Immune System

The immune system, a conglomerate of elements including specialized blood cells and the lymphatic system that runs throughout the body, protects us from disease. When a foreign invader such as a virus or bacterium tries to penetrate the body's defenses, an alarm goes off in the lymphatics that triggers the production of many different white blood cells. *Macrophages*, like little white knights, swamp the invader and knock him out; *T-cells* alert *B-cells* to produce *antibodies* to fight the infection that's set in.

IMMUNITY AND SLEEP. Is it possible that an enhanced sex life, which increases serotonin production but circulates the neurotransmitter freely throughout brain and body, could serve as a cure for insomnia?

Think about how well you sleep after feeling sexually satisfied. Chemically, you are in an optimal balance of blood and lymph chemicals that tell portions of the brain to shut down for several hours. You also have an appropriate level of melatonin (the hormone that regulates dark and light awareness) and of serotonin, a neurotransmitter that helps to promote well-being.

IMMUNITY AND TOUCH. Just a touch of a hand can change immune function. Whether it's a massage, laying-on-of-hands, petting an animal, or dancing cheek to cheek, we are deeply affected by skin on skin. When you are taking care of another person, you cannot do so without touching them almost constantly. The same is true of partners who seem bound to one another—there is always some physical link between them, whether it's just the casual touch of a hand on a shoulder or sitting with legs touching. The power of touch can keep us sane.

The very famous study on touch by Harry Harlow has been duplicated many times. In this experiment, Harlow took monkey babies away from their mothers and gave half the group a surrogate made of wire and cloth. The monkeys with the surrogate mother they could touch and groom grew up strong and sound of mind and body.

The monkeys who had no mother to hold onto, however, fought with each other over turf, refused to eat, and went mad without the initial life experience of touch.

Studies that came after Harlow went further in their investigation of this strange mechanism of touch deprivation. Dr. James Prescott and others have shown that if you deprive a laboratory animal of tactile and movement stimulation, it will exhibit abnormal social and emotional behavior.

The more we touch and hold our own children, the healthier their emotional brain centers will be—and the better chance they'll have in later life for learning to make strong affectional bonds of their own.

Current research in China and Japan reveals that it's not just the laying on of hands that makes the difference. In Chinese medicine, the life force we all possess is known as *chi*. Our own internal *chi* energy can relieve us of tension if we learn to practice structured breathing exercises (see Chapter Ten). But highly advanced practitioners can use their *chi* in a therapeutic way, much as biofeedback or acupuncture is used. The "touch" of this field of energy has been shown to inhibit the production of tumors in experimental mice in a laboratory, to accelerate the healing process of soft-tissue sports injuries, and to improve the prognosis of individuals suffering migraines, whiplash, and loss of cognitive function.

This type of therapeutic touch has not been widely investigated in the United States, but Chinese researchers explain the phenomenon in this way: External *chi* healers modulate the electromagnetic field around another body with their own life force. As the healer's *chi* accesses an injury or illness, it gets stronger in proportion to the need of the patient. Just as your own neurotransmitters jump across nerve synapses to offer information to your affected organs, so does *chi* energy transfer from one neurological system to another.

When you and your lover touch, you are exchanging more than the warmth of your hands and bodies. You are melding the life force that keeps you both going and enhancing it.

How a Good Sex Life Boosts Your Immunity

There appears to be a strong connection between immunity and sex. What we perceive of as a good sex life—and this is different for everyone—can make us more resistant to disease and stress. The arousal, desire, excitement and physical release of sexual activity enhances the natural abilities of the immune system to ward off illness. With a strong system, you are able to fight foreign antigens that threaten the body, and you can recover from illness more quickly when it does attack.

Now let's look at elements we get from our sexuality that have an impact on stress reduction and a protective immune system:

- lack of loneliness
- strong support system (good relationships can increase T-cell counts)
- exercise, which triggers lots of beta-endorphin activity in the brain
- positive attitude, also triggers endorphin response
- lowering of depression
- an ability to relax in the face of many obligations or upsets

- better "quality" sleep
- lots of touching
- being challenged
- having a commitment to something meaningful
- feeling in control

The two really coincide. Your sexuality can go a long way to enhance healing and create an environment where your immune system can function optimally.

Your Body's Sensory Organs and Genitals

Your body is rich in "feelers" that allow you to see, hear, touch, taste, smell, and experience life. But your sensory organs and your genitals derive their awareness from all the systems discussed earlier. You could not smell, for example, if your olfactory nerves didn't transmit a message to your brain.

If you are attuned to your lover's odor, you know there is nothing else like it in the world. Eskimos, of course, are one up on the rest of us with their custom of rubbing noses, just to get a whiff of their partner. There are certain dialects in Southern India where you ask your beloved, "give me a smell," instead of "give me a kiss." Meat eaters who live in hot climates or wear dark clothing are reputed to smell stronger than vegetarians who live in cool climates and wear light clothes. And each emotion we feel also changes our scent—just as fear can bring on a sharp odor, so joy and sexual interest can make us smell exciting and mysterious.

The smells of sex are incredibly distinctive—the odor of our cum, sweat, and saliva have a unique imprint. The skin and hair of each individual has its own attractant—all mixed up, of course, with the soap you wash with, the cologne you wear, and the materials that go into your clothing.

Those who are missing a sense—a blind or deaf individual, for example—tend to make up their lacks with particular strengths in other areas. If you can't see your lover, you can develop an exquisitely refined sense of touch. The skin, then, becomes an even more important sexual organ. And the mouth and tongue, with their dual ability to stimulate and taste, give us pathways into pleasure that must be explored to be enjoyed. When you whet your appetite for sex, there's no way back—you have to indulge your sense of taste and relish the whole banquet, from soup to nuts, from kisses to cunnilingus.

The genitals have been given such enormous weight in sexual influence in the past that I hesitate to downplay them. But really, a penis, vagina, clitoris, and nipples wouldn't do much for us without the stimulation of various hormones and neurotransmitters, adequate blood flow, appropriate skin contact, and the right frame of mind. The story of how these organs give us such incredible pleasure is discussed in Chapter Eleven in the section called "Questions and Answers About Orgasm."

The Mind—Your Most Powerful Sex Organ

I think, therefore I am. The desire to have a sexual encounter, the eagerness for a particular lover, the urge to be touched or touch in any particular way is derived from the mind. But where in the mind? How can we chart our libido, and figure out how much of our sexual interest comes from raging hormones, and how much is centered in limbic and cerebral cortex activity?

We feel a lot of things as sexual beings:

- We are moody and don't want to be touched.
- We want to be loved unequivocally.
- We are anxious that we won't measure up or that we won't be loved as much as we love.
- We remember a past experience with a lover and shiver as though it were happening all over again, actually feeling the touch of hands on us.
- We are greedy for power and control.
- We are afraid of being manipulated.
- We experience what should be pleasure, but instead feel pain, and vice versa.

The mind is the body's most powerful sexual organ. The thought of your lover kissing you can cause a rush and tingling over your entire body. An imagined fantasy about a sexual experience you've never had but crave deeply can make you delirious with anticipation. There's really no great trick to visualization—what you must do is give yourself the time and privacy to create scenarios in enormous detail. See the bed, hear the music, smell the flowers outside the window, touch the smooth sheets in your mind. Then add your lover. The memory of exactly what you did with your lover the last time, or the desire for what you'd like to do next time sharpens your mental skills and enhances your sexuality. There are those who can trigger an orgasm just from conjuring up an erotic mental scene.

Social Expectations

You aren't a sexual island. Rather, you are part of a social system that offers you groundwork and support for whatever you do. Each of us lives in a particular community at a particular time in the history of the world. Our attitudes and values (see Chapter Four) which come from family, friends, the media, the "experts," and our own good conscience, are formulated early in life and, it is hoped, evolve as we grow and develop.

Certain social obligations are laid upon us which we can meet or not meet, depending on how independent we are:

Do you have to link up with a person of the right sex, race, religion, species? Our society has paired heterosexual individuals for a very long time—only now are openly homosexual couples demanding their right to be together. Homosexual union, while barely tolerated in sophisticated communities, has caused such fury throughout most of our country that people who have "come out" sometimes fear for their lives. Is this any way to expect society to run? The prejudice and fear of gay couples is of course emblematic of all fears about the unknown or the uncommon. Couples of different races and until very recently, religions, have been stoned with the same vicious, jagged rocks.

Do you have to have a mate? People started pairing up centuries ago, and they've persisted in these joint ventures to the present day. Our society expects us to make a match at some time in our lives. But why do we have to be joined to another? Many individuals are quite happy alone, or are never able to find a suitable or compatible mate. Their sexual life may be masturbatory, sequential (a series of lovers), or nonexistent. And this is their prerogative.

Can you have sex with a friend? The movie *When Harry Met Sally* brings home the message about our cultural expectation to keep friendship free of sexual attachment. Yet some of the best friendships turn into partnerships or marriages, and some of the worst marriages take place between people who are not friends to begin with.

Do you have to sit by the phone and wait? How much power do you want in a relationship? How much are you allowed? Sometimes we act with a partner the way we think we're "supposed" to act. Sometimes we hold back, desiring to be pursued. The silence we invoke can be much more powerful than a needy demand for attention. But because sexual relationships, turn often on who wields power and how, this holding back can poison the best of matches.

All these elements—the biological, mental, emotional, and social—have an impact on our sexuality. But we don't have to split them up. As a matter of fact, we can't, because they're all part of one great system.

Dividing and Recombining Mind, Body, and Spirit

Look at the way the myriad influences on our sexuality come together in the diagram on the following page. The little shaded area in the middle is the culmination of all the elements that make us sexual beings. If scientists could dissect this piece of the action, they might be able to come up with extraordinary answers about mind and body.

The Power of Psychoneuroimmunology— Science of Self-healing

The burgeoning field of *psychoneuroimmunology* examines the inherent bonding of body and mind by studying the relationships among behavior, the brain, and the endocrine and immune systems. This field of study, developed by Robert Ader, Ph.D., a psychologist at the University of Rochester School of Medicine and Dentistry, offers us a new way of looking at the collaborative efforts of the various body systems. It is as if each cell of the body had within it a tiny mind and all cellular function proceeded as though controlled by its individual systems.

Humans respond to stimuli in ways that seem incomprehensible on first glance, but are pretty easy to understand if you think

Influences on Sexuality

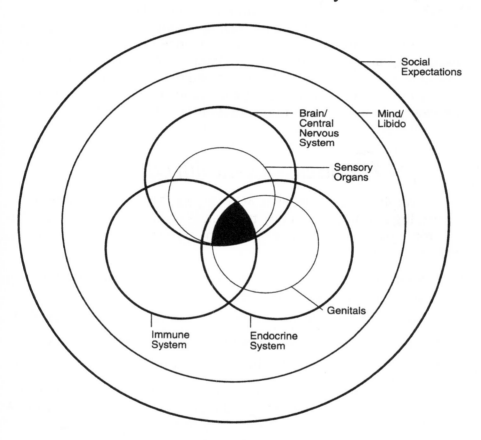

about the princinen didn't do so well. The candidates in the study
exposed to a if they were single or divorced. But this makes a lot
may be scnce women tend to carry the burden of the social, emo-
for disuomestic and childcare responsibilities in marriage. When
ecome overly involved in doing everything for everyone—and
sienting it—they can become depressed and even succumb to various illnesses.

REPAIRING THE DAMAGE: HOW TO GET STRESS UNDER CONTROL

If being tense is a prescription for being more susceptible
to illness, it stands to reason that relaxation would make you
healthier. In studies done on people with AIDS, a disease
where the immune system may shut down completely, it was
found that guided imagery techniques actually raised T-cell
counts. If you're depressed and feel hopeless, you will under-
go neuroendocrine and nervous system changes that put you
at risk for a compromised immune system. However, when
you can clear your mind by putting yourself into a meditative
state, and when you can develop a more positive attitude
toward your situation, you are increasing the activity of
restorative, protective T- and B-cells.

Robert Thayer, author of *The Biopsychology of Mood and Arousal*,
points out that the very same stress may hit you in entirely different
ways, depending on your mood. When you're aroused by stress, you
could feel very tense depending on what else is going on in your life.
Or you could feel very energized, as though stress were just what you
needed. Your mood may fluctuate between *tension* and *energy* on a
daily, weekly or yearly basis.

All of us experience periods of high tension and low energy—in
other words, you can be exhausted from getting terribly angry at
your partner. Many depressed people feel restless all the time, as
though they have to keep moving, keep doing just to stay functional.
But if we're healthy, we can work on finding times of high energy

and low tension—as when we've begun a relationship that gives us great pleasure and mutual satisfaction.

You may be concerned about whether this exultant relationship will continue, but that worry may appear challenging and exciting to you. If you regard this stress as though it were a gift, your mind will protect your body from harm.

What's Gender Got to Do with It?

As if all these things weren't enough influence on our sexuality, there is one more factor. It is usually mentioned first in sex books, but I mention it last, because, in my opinion, our society has given it far more emphasis than is healthy.

Are you male or female? Are you erotically aroused by males or females? Do you wish to play a male or female role when engaged in sexual activity with males or females? Were you born fixed with a certain affiliation, or can you change it if you want to?

Gender and then sexual orientation are at issue. Let's take these two apart to understand our maleness and femaleness—or the cross-over of the two—a little better.

Despite our chromosomes that divide us as males and females (XY for boys, XX for girls), we all start out physiologically as females in the womb. It is not until the fifth or sixth week of life that the gonads really kick in and become ovaries (female) or testes (male). There are abnormal chromosomal mixes (an extra X or a missing X, for example) that change the picture as well, but these are extremely rare.

But the male isn't technically a male yet, not until the seventh to twelfth week of life, when the male hormones—androgens—start being secreted by the testes. The penis itself doesn't develop until late in the second or early in the third trimester of pregnancy—in the absence of testosterone, the external genitals feminize and develop into a vagina, clitoris, and labia.

Where testosterone for the male and estrogen and progesterone for the female seem really significant, however, is at the brain level—they seem to influence the hypothalamus (where the pleasure center is located, remember) and organize a process that's called "sex-typing of the brain." This happens some time before we turn three years old.

So it isn't just chromosomes that determine gender, it's hormones as well.

Parents treat boys and girls differently because—as hard as we try—they are different. Males tend to be larger, so parents tend to bounce them around more and handle them more aggressively; girls tend to respond better to visual stimuli and social interaction, so parents make more eye contact with them. The behaviors we do that indicate our maleness or femaleness are further rewarded by a parent who expects certain behavior in their "sweet little girl" or "strong, feisty boy." And so it goes. All those messages we get that relate to aggressiveness and passivity, to directness and coyness, to which parts of our bodies it's okay to show in public, help to shape our gender identity.

When do we really make a sexual "choice"? Can we make it? Those who say that homosexuality is an abnormality have been shouted down by those who say it's genetic and hormonal. There is ample evidence to indicate that if we aren't born with a sexual orientation, we are certainly acclimatized to it in our earliest years. There are fetal, metabolic, hormonal, neural, familial, and social factors at play, and it would be impossible to divide them up or make one the deciding factor.

Luckily, we all become experts in gender by playing doctor and exploring our own genitals in the toddler and preschool years. There is nothing fixed about our sexuality—our fantasies indicate that our interest floats all over the map. What turns you on as a teenager may change radically by midlife. Kinsey felt that humans change sexually along the lifespan, but most orient themselves on one pole or another, with variations in between, on a bar graph that ranges from exclusively heteroerotic (1) to exclusively homoerotic (6) with small percentages of any given population at 1 or 6. We all may range around the 2 or 5 or even 3 or 4, in the right situations. Look what Kinsey says on the next page about our sexuality scale.

The Benefits of Changing—Or Updating— Your Sexual Orientation

Our concept of sexual orientation is often life-long, but it really doesn't have to be that way. If you feel stuck in the wrong camp— as do many in our society—you can end up with some awful problems. Our real orientation, or direction toward the type of person we're attracted to, can make itself known in the space of time it

The Kinsey Sexuality Scale

Exclusive hetero-sexuality	Predominant hetero-sexuality with incidental homo-sexuality	Predominant hetero-sexuality	Ambi-sexuality	Predominant homo-sexuality with more than incidental hetero-sexuality	Predominant homo-sexuality with incidental hetero-sexuality	Exclusive homo-sexuality

takes us to make eye contact across a room. Someone who considered himself a tried-and-true heterosexual may in fact be startled and terrified when he happens to hug another man at a party and finds that he has an erection. This doesn't necessarily mean he has become homosexual, yet it can be a frightening revelation to see that he can, under the right circumstances, be attracted to both sexes.

Sexual orientation is not graven in stone. According to sexologist William Stayton, we are born "pansexual," with the ability to gravitate toward any and all elements of the universe—we could find erotic pleasure in a leaf, a ray of sunlight, a dog. Next, we learn to be turned on by ourselves, and finally, when we can approach the outside world, we are drawn to others. Stayton uses a different model than Kinsey, which is shown on the next page.

And many people, after years of one exclusive orientation, find themselves with shifting desires. Some say they were born and raised heterosexual, even though they knew all along this was not their true orientation at all. It may take a huge life change to push the individual with a homosexual preference to admit that this is what he or she was intended to be.

It's very frightening for most people to recognize their potential for attraction to both genders. But attraction is as ephemeral as lik-

Female Reproductive Organs and Genitals

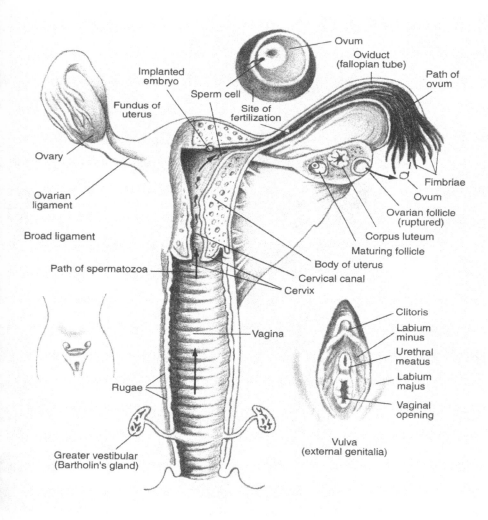

Ovum
Oviduct (fallopian tube)
Path of ovum
Implanted embryo
Sperm cell
Fundus of uterus
Site of fertilization
Ovary
Fimbriae
Ovarian ligament
Ovum
Ovarian follicle (ruptured)
Broad ligament
Corpus luteum
Maturing follicle
Path of spermatozoa
Body of uterus
Cervical canal
Cervix
Clitoris
Vagina
Labium minus
Urethral meatus
Labium majus
Rugae
Vaginal opening
Greater vestibular (Bartholin's gland)
Vulva (external genitalia)

Side View of Female Internal Reproductive Organs

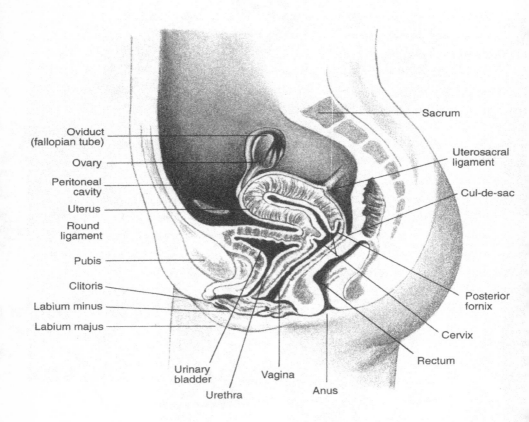

Following the body around toward the rear, the next structure is the *perineum*, the space of flesh between the vagina and the *anus*, the opening to the rectum in back. The euphoniously named *mound of Venus* is the fleshy covering of the pubic bone at the front.

All the rest of a female's reproductive tract is internal. The vagina leads to the mouth of the *uterus*, which is called the *cervix*. This structure is an amazing little opening, which can stretch wide enough to permit a baby to pass, yet is so tight in the nonpregnant woman that the string of an IUD can fit snugly inside it. The uterus, a pear-shaped muscular organ just on top of the bladder, is a potential home for a developing fetus, and it is lined with tissue called the *endometrium*. This tissue gets alternately thicker and thinner during the course of a month under the influence of the fluctuating ovarian hormones, *estrogen* and *progesterone*. At the end of each monthly cycle, the endometrium is shed during your *menses*.

Your reproductive glands, the *ovaries*, sit in the abdominal cavity and are held in place by ligaments that attach them to the uterus and the body wall. From each ovary extends a *Fallopian tube*, which ends in little graceful fingerlike structures called *fimbriae*. After ovulation, the egg is carried away from the ovary by peristalsis and the sweeping action of cilia that line the tubes.

If you are a man, your penis is about two to four inches long when not erect. (See the diagram on page 52.) It is composed of several structures: the *glans* or head on top of which is the *prepuce*, the loose fold of skin at the end of the penis. Uncircumcised men retain the entire prepuce, or foreskin. The *frenulum* is the fleshy sensitive ridge on the underside and just behind it, and the *shaft* runs up the length of the penis. Inside the shaft are three columns of tissue threaded with blood vessels which become engorged (and therefore erect) during arousal—the *corpus cavernosa* are the two columns on either side of the penis and the *corpus spongiosum* is the column in between which contains the *urethra*. This tube carries the urine from the bladder to the opening at the end of the glans.

Now we move on to the *scrotal sac* hanging behind the penis. Inside this protective sac, the two *testes* are couched together, one usually hanging slightly below the other. These are the reproductive organs of the male body, corresponding to the ovaries in the female body. On top of each testis is the *epididymis*, a long coiled tube that is the first portion of the complicated duct system of the male reproductive tract. The *vas deferens* is also part of this system. It is a

Side View of Male Internal Reproductive Organs

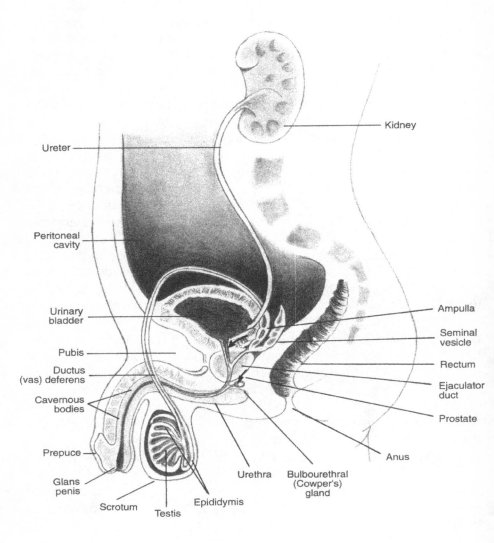

straight tube starting at the epididymis and extending into the abdominal cavity, around the bladder and down to the base of the *prostate gland* and finally to the *seminal vesicle*. This is the important duct that carries the sperm from the epididymis to the *ejaculatory duct*. The prostate gland is a small, walnut-shaped structure behind the bladder that releases a milky, alkaline substance that keeps the sperm at its proper pH level. Your partner can give you a great deal of pleasure by putting a finger about one inch up inside your *anus* and stimulating this gland during sex.

During the arousal process, as the corpora swell with blood, the pressure on all the surrounding structures cause a release of *semen* into the urethra. Semen is the viscous white fluid containing the spermatozoa, which is emitted via the muscular contractions of the testes, epididymides, seminal vesicles, and prostate gland. When you are about to come, these contractions draw the testes up against the body. At this point, the conjoined tubes perform an intricate shutdown process so that no urine can escape into the urethra at the same time as it fills with spermatozoa. The *Cowper's glands* just below the prostate on either side of the urethra secrete an alkaline substance that coats the lining of the urethra to neutralize its acidity in preparation for the arriving spermatozoa.

Now that you can see in black and white how your genital and reproductive area is built, it's time to examine the real-life structures.

EXERCISE
A Self-exploration Before the Mirror

Spend at least twenty minutes naked in front of a mirror, getting acquainted with your body parts. Examine all of them—don't skip any. Women, place a mirror on the floor and squat down over it so that you can see everything. As one gynecologist friend of mine so aptly stated, "If more people would spend more time looking in the mirror at their genitals and less time at their faces, we'd have a lot less sexually transmitted disease and a lot more comfort with our sexuality."

It is always a revelation to see this miracle of form and structure, each organ and tissue exactly suited to its purpose. If you know your genitals intimately when they are healthy, you have a barometer for their general normal appearance. This way, if you notice any changes, lumps, discolorations, and so on, you can get to a physician quickly and determine the source of the trouble.

Borrow the Mind of a Child
to Explore Your Body

Kids aren't inhibited about what they do and how they react. They make funny faces, stick out their tongues, jump and skip, and act like they were made of rubber one minute, of steel the next. This is what I'd like you to try. Sex is a way for adults to play with one another, but if you aren't comfortable fooling around by yourself, it will be hard to share the fun with a partner.

To really appreciate the brilliance of the physical housing you've been designated to live in, you have to start with a beginner's mind—that is, you have to look at yourself as though you'd never seen a human body before.

You could not walk, talk, eat, laugh, cry, or sleep if you did not have the biology, mentality, emotionality and spirituality you were born with. The functions you perform are as simple as swallowing food and as complex as being able to understand another's pain.

Sit right where you are and examine your hand, that very important grasping, feeling organ with its wiggling fingers and opposable thumb. And you have two of them! Get up now and think about your balance that allows you to stand on your two feet and not fall over. Try going up a flight of stairs, then coming down. Think about the muscles that pull and push your legs as they work alternately to get you to your goal.

Make your jaws open and let a few words come out. Then a sound that has some meaning to you. Experiment a little and see just what this vocal equipment can do. You may reach sounds high enough to shatter glass or deep enough to vibrate the floor.

Isn't this a revealing exercise? You see how much you take for granted every day. This body, filled with energy, glowing with strength and vitality, is your gift. You can keep it to yourself, you can lend it to a friend, you can mix and match its power and fragility in the beautiful act that joins it to that of another. For those brief moments in time when we hold another's body inside ours or are held by them, we can truly fathom why ancient societies viewed sexual intimacy as a spiritual union. When we join our energy to that of a beloved, we are expanding them and ourselves simultaneously.

Seven Exercises to Enhance Your Sexuality

Here is a set of pleasure exercises for you to try. There's no sex involved, just pleasure. You need these exercises to prepare you for those in later chapters, so don't skip them just because you want to get to the sex part! These are particularly important for those who have survived sexual or emotional abuse which has caused them to dislike their bodies, and for those who have made unconventional sexual choices. These people may have spent a great deal of time covering up their interest in the body so that no one would notice how different they were. The point of the exercises is to play and have fun. They will give you the opportunity to revel in your unique God-given body.

EXERCISE
Body Basics

1. Stand on one foot with your eyes closed for as long as you can. Think about only one thought at a time, let it go, then select a new one.

2. Take off your clothes without using your hands. If this is too hard at first, you may use your palms but not your fingers.

3. Spread your fingers and toes as wide as you can, then interlace them. Breathe deeply in this posture for one minute.

4. Block your ears with cotton and turn in a circle one way ten times, then the other. Start slowly, then build up speed. You should do this on a soft surface, in case you fall down.

5. Visit a playground alone, or with your partner. Use all the playground equipment. Be sure you get in some climbing, some falling, some sliding, some pushing and pulling, and getting in and out of tight spaces.

6. Experiment with different types of breathing, both alone and with a partner. If you practice coordinated breathing, you are synchronizing more than just your desire for each other—you are aligning both your cardiovascular and respiratory systems. This type of practice enhances the ability to take sex to a different level (see Chapter Thirteen to learn about Tantric and Taoist sexuality).

Inhale through your mouth, exhale through nose and mouth until your repetitions are even and comfortable. Then try inhaling slowly, holding your breath for a count of ten, then exhaling slowly. Coordinate with your partner.

Challenge each other with different breathing combinations, fast and slow, held and free. Imagine breathing into different body organs—send the breath to your head, your limbs, your back and spinal column, your genitals.

Take turns inhaling and exhaling into each other's mouths—the sensation will be extraordinary if you have never done this before. Make sure one person is the giver, the other the receiver. Check with your partner to see that you are not giving or taking so much oxygen that it causes dizziness.

7. Sense your body's reaction to different fabrics. Take your clothes off, lie down and prepare to be quiet for twenty minutes. Then take a piece of velvet, silk, linen, burlap, wool, chamois and cotton and touch them to different parts of you. Do this gently, roughly, teasingly, and so on.

EXERCISE
How Well Do You Know Your Partner's Body and Mind?

Do You Know What Your Partner Wants? A want is something you'd like (as opposed to a need, which is something you absolutely must have to survive). When you get what you want, you tend to be satisfied, unless your expectation was radically different from possibility. We rarely balance our desires against reality. How do your sexual wants measure up to your partner's?

Answer yes or no to the following

	I Want (Y/N)	My Partner Wants (Y/N)
Frequent sexual relations		
Experimentation		
Mutual masturbation		
Fantasy		
Sex out of bed		

	I Want (Y/N)	My Partner Wants (Y/N)
Sex with toys		
Sex at different times of day		
Variety		
Open talk		
Oral sex		
Anal sex		
Light bondage		
Guiltless masturbation		
Live with a lover		
Extend pleasure before intercourse		
More nudity		
More cuddling and touching		
Orgasm		

SECRET AND SHARED COMMUNICATIONS. We tell our partners certain things and withhold others. We would be greatly surprised to know that what we consider strange, weird, or kinky, others might think of as totally routine, and vice versa. Make a list of sexual experiences, feelings, ideas, impulses, and desires you have shared with a partner and those you have kept secret. Then switch lists. You may find that some of your closed items are open for your partner. The communication process may help both of you bring more items into the shared column.

WHAT DO YOU KNOW? This quiz is primarily for heterosexual lovers. Gays and lesbians are not handicapped by having to understand the anatomy, desires, and preferences of their partner, because they generally have the same or similar ones.

MEN:

- Do you know that most women are turned on by talk? If you begin by telling her just what you find exciting about her, or what you'd like to do when you're alone together, you may have her panting. If you start by pulling her close and kissing and touching, you may lose her.

- Do you know that women don't always like their clitoris stimulated first? And some like just the sides, not the top. Ask before you dive in roughly. This applies to oral sex as well—a lot of tongue pressure directly on the clitoris can hurt. Try to nibble, suck, kiss, and lick the entire vulva—labia, vagina, and clitoris, alternating areas and touches.

- Do you know that most women feel next to nothing through the vaginal walls, which aren't really plentiful in nerve endings. The excitement of intercourse is usually a combination of elements—stimulation of clitoris, breasts, G-spot, anus, mouth, and the wash of desire in general gives most women a lot more than an object alone (penis or vibrator) thrusting in and out.

- Do you know that women usually want you to continue stimulation after they begin to orgasm? If you have your hand, tongue, penis, or anything else inside your partner when she begins to come, *by all means leave it there and keep the stimulation going.* If you neglect to do this, your partner may lose the orgasm or certainly not experience the fullness of it.

- Do you know that some women are turned off by making love during their period and some are really turned on by it? Ask. The same may be true during pregnancy and when she's nursing.

- Do you know that women typically don't lubricate much during their period? This doesn't mean they aren't aroused—but you will need some saliva or commercial water-based lubricant such as Replens, Astroglide, or KY Jelly so that neither of you is uncomfortable.

- Do you know that women don't always prize the man who can "go forever"? It is a cause for great macho celebration for most men to be able to say they can stay hard for an hour without coming, but it can be a real turn-off to a woman, who may just be tired and disinterested (and sore) after twenty minutes of vigorous thrusting.

- Do you know that a woman's nipples may be terribly sensitive, particularly before and during her period, and that the borderline between pleasure and pain may be quite thin? Be gentle with sucking and biting nipples unless told otherwise. Rimming them with your tongue, very gently and teasingly, is the most wonderful course of action.

- Do you know that some women may balk at oral sex because they're afraid you will find their odor offensive? It's important to assure a woman that she smells and tastes great to you.

- Being nervous about anal sex may also have to do with odor, but will in most cases relate to the pain factor—a lubricant is always needed. Be sure you wash your penis after anal sex if you are going to have vaginal sex afterward to prevent the transmission of bacteria from one orifice to the other.

- Do you know that menopause need not have any bearing on a woman's sex drive? (She loses estrogen at menopause, but it's her testosterone that boosts her libido.) The lack of estrogen does make for a dry vagina, however, so she may not lubricate as easily and may need a longer period of time—and a water-based lubricant—to become aroused.

- Hysterectomy or tubal ligation (female sterilization) may not influence a woman's sex drive at all—she will simply need time to heal from her operation before being comfortable with penetration in the case of a hysterectomy. If she does experience a decline in libido, it is due to a decrease in her circulating androgens after the procedure. This problem can be treated with medication. The ligation is performed endoscopically, through a small incision near the bellybutton, and the healing process will involve slightly sore stomach muscles. In both cases, the psychological healing from the loss of a woman's reproductive potential may take far longer than the physical.

- Do you know that flattery is a great boost to the sexual experience? Most women are insecure about the way their bodies look and feel, and a word of praise can never go amiss. To say "you have the most beautiful legs in the world and I love to run my fingers down them" can be an enormous turn-on.

WOMEN:

- Do you know that there is no difference in sensitivity between men who are and are not circumcised? They both feel just as much at the head of the penis. The only difference is that the uncircumcised man must be slightly more careful about washing the genital area after sex because bacteria can become caught within the folds of the foreskin.

- Do you know that your partner cannot accidentally urinate into your vagina during sex? The duct that carries urine from the bladder down the urethra closes during sex.

- Do you know that certain men's testicles seem to be more joined together, as if they were one testicle? This doesn't mean there's anything wrong.

- Do you know that men can urinate sitting down? And frequently do, when they're having a bowel movement.

- Do you know that vasectomy does not lower a man's sex drive? The amount of ejaculate may be slightly less in some vasectomized men.

- Did you know that a vasectomy does not "take" right away? There may still be some sperm left in the semen for up to sixteen weeks after the surgery, because whatever was in the vas deferens prior to the operation must be ejaculated first. Use some form of contraception during this time.

- Did you know that the ability to have an erection, orgasm, and ejaculation does not mean that a man is necessarily able to conceive a child? Fertility or infertility has nothing to do with potency.

- Do you know that erectile dysfunction—the inability to achieve or maintain an erection—does not mean that your partner doesn't want you or doesn't find you exciting? The loss of erection can stem from many causes, physical and psychological, and it certainly shouldn't keep the two of you from making love. An erection is only one pleasuring stimulus—for both of you—amid a whole host of others.

- Do you know that some men get off on having you hold their testicles when you have oral sex and some don't like it at all? Ask first.

- Do you know that your partner's penis is incredibly sensitive after he has come, and he may not even want you to touch or kiss it for five or ten minutes afterward?

- Do you know that some men really love it if you stick a lubricated finger up their anus when they are coming because it can greatly enhance orgasm? But others find it invasive. Always ask.

- Do you know that it's very common for your partner to be unable to enjoy himself during sex? He may be so concentrated on giving you an orgasm, he completely negates his own pleasure. You can spend some time just giving to him. Tell him, it turns me on to turn you on—so lie back and enjoy it!

- Do you know that your partner may be having a wonderful time even if he doesn't make a sound? Men are more inhibited than women when it comes to letting go and screaming or moaning.

- Do you know that your partner may enjoy different sensations during oral sex? You can kiss the head of his penis, stimulating the frenulum (the ridge in back of and beneath the head) with your tongue, you can move your mouth up and down on the shaft, or if you don't have a strong gag reflex, you can take his whole penis into your mouth. Some people are able to "deepthroat," actually open their throat completely to accommodate the length of the shaft.

- Do you know that your partner may experience pain during intercourse if you are not sufficiently lubricated? Saliva or a commercial water-based lubricant is a great idea for couples of any age. A more uncommon problem that could cause him pain is the bending or bowing of his erect penis. This is the result of a medical condition called Peyronie's disease.

- Do you know that it's no reflection on you if your partner turns to look at another woman? You might recognize the fact that you do the same thing, but perhaps more subtly. Men are reputed to crave variety and novelty in sexual partners more than women—but there's no evidence of this. They may scour the field because of the peer pressure they encountered in adolescence when all the guys were checking out all the girls. Most normal men have no intention of running off with the person they're checking out. It's a visual stimulation thing only. But most *must* check her out.

Learning about one another's desires can help you learn more about your own. You may be astounded at facts, fears, and feelings that you've forgotten or kept under wraps for a long time.

4

How
to Achieve a
Healthy Attitude
Toward Sex

*H*annah told me she kept her life in ice cube trays. Each event was a separate, self-contained cube, and she could take them out at will to defrost and use. The image might have come originally from the cold, restrictive nature of her family. Sex didn't exist for her parents, a strict Southern Baptist alcoholic father and a terrified "good-girl" mother, or for her three older sisters. Hannah, unlike the rest of her family, however, was not frozen through and through. She had started to melt in early puberty when she began to masturbate and had what she describes as "a virginal sense of strong self-love."

She defrosted one of those ice cubes when she married her first husband, the boy she clung to out of infatuation. He filled her with such a sense of wonder when he sucked her breasts that she said she had to keep him around. Her second husband took out another ice cube. He enthralled her verbally, telling her she was wonderful in so many ways and enough times so that she could believe it. A quick thaw for a third cube came with the first woman she slept with, her supervisor in the school district where she taught.

Hannah is now in her early fifties and has been with the same female lover for fifteen years. She never used the word lesbian in our conversations, perhaps because it's a word that implies "outsider" or "different," and she doesn't feel that way. The kind of sexuality she can express with a woman comes from a different part of her, a part that might have been suspended in the ice for years, just waiting to be tapped. There was no particular continuum between the way she expressed herself physically and psychically with men and with women. Each was valid and separate for her.

But the really essential ice cube never would have melted if she had been fixed in the old attitudes her family bequeathed to her. If she had modeled herself on the expectations of the last generation, she would never have found happiness.

Healing Your Sexual Attitudes

You cannot be a healthy sexual person unless your perceptions about your sexuality and others' is comfortable to you and fits you just right. You can't act like a joyous individual if you carry the fears and superstitions from your early years on your back. If you are still lugging around old garbage from your past or holding on to values that don't match your own, there is no way you can accept yourself, your needs and feelings. If you can change your attitude, however, you have a great chance at healing your psyche, your emotional life, and your personality. This healing process, by the way, isn't a difficult one for most people. It requires an open mind and a sensitive awareness of your typical reactions to situations. When you see that by adjusting your attitude, you can relax and enjoy yourself, the rewards will reinforce your new behaviors.

The pervasiveness of your sexuality in your life is something you are just now getting in touch with—so this is the time to sensitize that touch. The fact that everything you encounter in life rebounds off your sexuality means that you must have your head on straight about what you think and feel is "right" to do.

If you were brought up to believe that homosexuals were sick and deranged, and you are a homosexual, you are going to have a lot of healing work to do inside and outside. You will not only have to confront the devils that hovered around your childhood, you will also have to challenge society's antipathy to who you are and what you do as you struggle to achieve sexual union with the person you've become.

If you're a heterosexual man and were brought up to believe that you had to "satisfy a woman every time," you may get furious at your partner if she doesn't come to your satisfaction. You can only heal if you accept the fact that you're not responsible for her orgasms, but only your own pleasure.

If you're a heterosexual woman and you learned early on that women only got into that conjugal bed for the purpose of pleasing a man, you are probably filled with rage every time you defer your own needs. You will heal only if you're able to tell yourself that you deserve to be touched well, with perception and kindness and just the right mix of suspense and clear definition.

Where Our Attitudes Toward Sex Come From

We all learned about sex from someone in charge. Either we were indoctrinated by parents, siblings, church, or school, or we heard rumors about it from friends or saw it plastered on billboards and TV. Possibly, we were influenced by one song or book that clicked with our fantasies. Just a few of us got to see it in the raw— but watching animals fornicate doesn't begin to approach the intricacies of human sexuality. If we dared to peer through a bedroom keyhole at six or eight and were stunned by the sights and sounds of our parents making love, we couldn't have assimilated what any of it meant. But still, those first impressions were lasting because they affected us when we weren't ready to combat their overwhelming stimulation.

Family Influence

We are so much a product of the way we were raised. Even if you never had the conversation with your parents that went, "sex is dirty unless you're married" (with the addition for boys, "but if you can get away with it, it's okay"), you surely must have picked up numerous messages along the way, just by watching your mom and dad interact. Children who never see their mother and father hugging and kissing, who are shoved out of the bathroom when their parents are naked, who are exposed to direct or covert expressions of homophobia or sexual abuse or sexual phobias of any kind will surely incorporate these horrors into their body of beliefs.

Cultural Influence

What we learn in our family setting is often culturally bound. For example, most African-American girls are taught that it's wrong to touch themselves, and this belief is reinforced even more than in Caucasian or Asian families. This puts a severe damper on useful tools for healthy sexuality, such as tampons for menstrual hygiene, diaphragms for contraception, and masturbation for pleasure. It can be difficult for an African-American woman to take charge of what goes on in the bedroom because it is expected that the man "takes care of business."

It's part of the Greek tradition, and also the tradition for certain Hispanic groups, for young men to select same-sex partners before they accept their traditional matrimonial obligations. But if you asked if they'd had any homosexual experiences, they'd be shocked. In their culture, this is not considered sexual deviation but, rather, experimentation.

Religious Influence

Sex and the devil have always been linked in the Judeo-Christian tradition. Although some faiths are urged to give pleasure to their mates (you can interpret this as sexual pleasure if you wish), others are told in no uncertain terms that if they aren't reproducing, they're sinning. The rules and regulations that governed man and woman in biblical days certainly had cultural import at the time; whether they pertain at all to what we do with our loved ones today is questionable. It's incredibly hard to get rid of this one—religion drummed so many terrible attitudes into our heads at such an impressionable age. It's not impossible to heal from these, but we must be willing to alter our attitude drastically and grant that God will love us for enjoying ourselves sexually. In good, healthy sex, we are doing unto others as we would have others do unto us—which is, you'll recall, the golden rule.

Peer Influence

If your friends do it, it's cool. If not, not. From our pals, we pick up a potpourri of mistaken, misshapen, and haphazard information about sex and love, mostly based on peer pressure and what the little kids heard from the bigger ones. This can be a liberating education for many who were held back sexually at home. Mark, a self-described "country boy," said he learned about sex when he was six or seven from running around the woods near his rural North Carolina home. "We'd play hide and seek a lot," he said. "It was boys and girls together, catching frogs, swinging on ropes over the swimming hole, building forts by the lake, and running around in the water. When we were really wet, we'd take those clothes off and run around in the pine grove. I think it was really erotic, seeing all the other kids like that, and by the time I was thirteen or so, we weren't just looking. A few of us would explore—natural curiosity—touching each others' genitals, then rubbing till it felt good."

Another big teacher is society. We get "expert opinions" from TV, radio, books, magazines, and our physicians if they deign to offer sexual advice (most don't). We get "everyone else's opinions" when we read the words, set in stone, by Gallup and Harris, of those millions around the country whose attitudes have relevance to us only in terms of numbers. If lots of people believe a certain thing, it must be so. Right?

Wrong. So many people who look to others to form their opinions have been brainwashed with the following epithets:

"Being coupled is right, everyone ought to have *someone*."

"Homosexuality is not only deviant but catching—stay away from *them*."

"A woman can't be too aggressive sexually or she'll scare a man off."

"It's okay for boys to fool around, but a girl's going to get a reputation if she does."

"You've got to use condoms when you're with new partners, but not with a boyfriend or girlfriend you really love."

Society's attitudes, ranging from totally dangerous, as in the idiotic prescription for protection sometimes and not at others, to bizarre proscriptions on gender roles and behavior to courtship, dating and coupling are rigid and difficult to question once they're in your system. Like a tapeworm, they wind themselves deeper into your gut, holding on for dear life.

False Beliefs About Sex and How to Change Them

We can heal our stunted beliefs as soon as we start to *think*. Sometimes, we cling to views because we've never questioned them. But if we take apart the attitude, it may be quite easy to see that it is based on nothing.

I encourage you to take your old irrational beliefs, examine them rigorously, and substitute new beliefs based on real—not imagined—information about sexual attitudes. Shake your mind up! Your mental health will improve dramatically as soon as you begin to reinforce your new beliefs with lots of practice. For example:

False belief #1: Sex is dirty unless it's in the context of marriage.

You may be married or unmarried and still hold to this old saw. To change your thoughts about sex, ask yourself what is actually different in the married and unmarried state. Unmarried people may be more open and giving to one another, more exploratory and interested in getting to know one another. Married people may perform "the act" as an obligation, regardless of their feelings about it. The "dirtiness" or raunchiness depends completely on the couple, married or unmarried.

New belief: Sex is appropriate—not dirty or clean—between two individuals who care about and respect one another.

False belief #2: "Men like big breasts; women like big penises."

It is interesting that this one has stuck around so long, but we may assume that it carries on the American tradition of "bigger is better." In fact, studies reveal that the majority of men state unequivocally that "more than a mouthful is wasted"; so many women have declared that a very large penis can be uncomfortable or even painful to accommodate.

New belief: Body parts and shapes are simply the accoutrements of one individual with many more facets than the physical. Since attraction is couched in dozens of elements that include personality, cultural expectation, common interests, availability, biochemical attractants, as well as physical attributes, how you're built only makes a difference to people you probably wouldn't be happy with in the long run anyway.

You can run this process on any belief you've got and turn it around. However, you must reinforce your new beliefs by taking them for trial runs and testing them out repeatedly. Only in this way can you effectively change the way you think about your sexuality.

Mark, whose wife Cynthia had been brought up in an extremely repressed household, said that "her background made her afraid to give her heart. But, probably as rebellion against her parents, she loved acting like a 'bad girl'; that's how she described it. We'd drive to the beach in our Landrover, and we'd go park somewhere—not always completely private. And there she'd be with her legs up in the air, having one orgasm after another. We did it in movie theaters, too," he added with a smile. Cynthia got a lot of practice, but never really changed her belief. "She just didn't feel right afterward about letting go so much, and she'd cry terribly for having given herself all that pleasure. And after she got breast cancer, she felt too tired most of the time to relate to me the way she really wanted to."

Yet Angela, a forty-eight-year-old woman who had been abused as a child, was really able to heal her terribly warped beliefs about her sexuality. "I believed for so long that I was a victim, so I did stuff to stay a victim. But finally, I saw that my sexual needs as an adult were different from those I'd been forced to commit to when I was a child. I did feel horny with my husband, James—we just fit; we actually went through one another when we made love. I was lousy to him for making me want him at first, because I thought it was wrong, based on everything I felt about my father. But James just kept accepting my shit. Finally, I saw I was hurting him like I'd been hurt. I didn't have to do that anymore. And when I realized that, sex got easier. It really started to be fun."

EXERCISE
Shedding More False Beliefs About Sex

Take apart the following irrational beliefs and replace them with logical facts. Seeing your sexuality from a broader perspective—what your mind, body, and spirit feels—will lead you to change your attitudes and abolish old myths.

False beliefs:

1. I must be a pervert if I want so much sex.

2. I must be repressed if I don't feel sexual.

3. After fifty, nobody's really interested in sex.

4. After you're married, the fun goes out of sex.

5. You shouldn't have sex during your period.

6. Masturbation takes away your interest in "real" sex.

7. The only real orgasm is a vaginal orgasm.

8. Women who dress provocatively are "asking for it."

9. You can't have sex after a colostomy.

10. Aphrodisiacs will make repressed people come.

When you read these, they appear to be ridiculous. And yet they are common beliefs that are hard to shake. Don't expect your new beliefs to come automatically—you are working against years of brain-washing.

How to Teach Boys and Girls About Sexual Stereotypes

I'm distressed that the women's and men's movements of the 1970s and 1990s have done virtually nothing to equalize the sexes. The decks are still stacked sexually from a very early age. The most liberated parents cringe at the idea of their macho little boy taking ballet lessons and their delicate little girl becoming a firefighter.

So what's considered normal? When boys join a sex posse and feel they have the right to rape their classmates, they're just feeling their oats. But what if girls did it? They'd be run out of town or locked up in a mental institution. Now here's a startling thought: What if children of both sexes were taught at an early age that sexual experimentation was great and good as long as it was consensual and a crime if it was forced? Ah, then, our society would be healing itself.

Think about an elementary school classroom. Early Brownie points go to girls who mature faster and stick with a task while little boys are still stuck on being loud and running in circles. However, the tables are turned in middle school, where the aggressive hand-raisers who jump right in to answer the question or volunteer for the assignment first are considered most likely to succeed. Girls, programmed in kindergarten to sit quietly, are at a great disadvantage here—unless they start "acting like boys."

It is difficult to buck society's attitudes on what men and women are allowed and not allowed to do. These days, it's okay for a teenage girl to invite a male to the prom, but she has to have guts to do it because clearly, she'll be in the minority. (She'll be even more in the minority if she invites another girl.) It's customary to see tough women in the boardroom, and yet, they are penalized for acting with the same no-nonsense manner outside the executive suite. A woman who is "too independent" is in many ways more an outsider than a man who is nurturing and empathic—because women want men to feel more (and be more like them), they reward a man who understands.

We are still bucking some very old stereotypes about what men and women are supposed to be and do. Our male–female choices these days are psychologically based, given the scientific evidence that women's brains and men's brains work differently in relationships. But so what, if *some* women really are more nurturing, more compassionate, more internal, and more love-centered? So what if *some* men are more direct and assertive, can concentrate on one subject at a time and are able to separate love and sex? Others are not built this way. Maybe *you* are not.

Let me make a valiant call for bucking society's expectations. What everybody else thinks may in fact be wrong! It is enormously hard to dance your own dance, but if it's good enough, it may catch on and you'll have more partners than you know what to do with. (And this time, you don't have to wait to be asked to fox trot.)

*S*plitting Sex and Love: Should You Do It If You Can?

We are still living under the curse of the old Romance tradition of the Middle Ages—the one that valued the *idea* of love over the *practice* of love. All these hundreds of years later, and we still buy into the romance claptrap of the soap opera and the Harlequin paperback. It is hard to grow up to be a passionate being if you believe you have to link souls for all eternity before you jump in the sack.

Yet, this is the kind of wrongheaded thinking that led so many of us into marriages without promise and doomed us to search constantly for that perfect individual who would arrive with our name (and only ours) engraved on his or her noble brow.

If you approach the idea of union with another—physical, mental, emotional, spiritual—as permissible only if you "love" the person, you may never be contented with what you get, because your ideals are so damned exacting.

No one in the world can meet all your standards and fulfill all your expectations. Why should a life partner be your lover, financial manager, gourmet chef, nurse, caretaker, parent, comedian, nurturing parent to your kids, dark soul, intellectual goad, and chief bottlewasher? We cannot be all things to all people.

The combination of longing to belong and wanting desperately to wrap things up quickly made many of us marry young and regret it soon after. The people we were in high school and college have changed irrevocably with the years, and many early matches can't survive that evolution. Even those marriages that took place in our thirties need to be reexamined ten or twenty years later, when both parties have both been grownups together for a long time.

In this age when divorce leaves you open to a rotten financial picture as well as a dangerous sexual marketplace, many people settle. "This is all I deserve," they say, and because they married for love, they figure the love has died, or maybe, if they're lucky, it'll come back when the kids leave the house.

This is absurd. There's no reason why we must always be partnered with the same person, or why we should be forbidden from feeling sexually about others. We certainly don't have to act on all our fantasies, but it's death to the soul to squelch them because they make us so guilty. Our sexual feelings cannot continue to be bound up in the craving for everlasting love.

It is possible for some people to achieve sexual pleasure with someone they don't love—naturally, the same precautions apply for physical contact in each case. Most of those I interviewed for this book claimed that they can't—or won't—do this. They must feel a real connectedness with an individual, which they term "love," before slipping between the sheets.

But others—more men than women—acknowledged that sure, they can "just have sex," and enjoy it, even if they never intend to see the one-night stand again. One man told me that he had known his first lover for only two hours before he decided to sleep with her. But he was certain that he was fond of her, and this was his reason for deciding to give up his virginity to her.

Let's look at both sets of attitudes for a moment. Is it possible that the people who claim to need "relatedness" are conning themselves in many cases? Perhaps they are simply convincing themselves that their partner cares enough to make it legit. And is it also conceivable that those who say they can enjoy "casual sex" wish to distance themselves from the incredible rush that takes place when we bond physically with another? By stating it would be just this one time and that it had nothing to do with caring deeply, they are protecting themselves from possible rejection.

The "love" we feel for a husband or wife, a child, a parent, and the men and women in our lives who have touched us deeply is simply not transferrable. Some single thread may run through all the relationships we consider important, but they are so individual as to be like different languages. As for sex, how wonderful that each partner, each time together, each orgasm is unique unto itself.

If sex and love have a meeting ground, and I think they do, it probably has to do with time. Time to learn what can and can't happen between two people. It doesn't have to be long term, it doesn't necessarily have to be monogamous as long as all precautions—emotional as well as physical—are used. It cannot exist in the hazy wish of a couple trying to pretend that they are joined at the hip to justify getting into bed together.

What I would wish for each healthy being on the planet is a network of adjunct friendships that might be sexual or might simply be platonic. If you had a great marriage, but discovered a passion for chess with a woman you also found terribly attractive, and you loved going to the theater with a man you were also drawn to, it would be okay. It would not create chaos in your world because you would have divided up the part of you that loved your spouse and enjoyed being sexual with your spouse, and the part of you eager to share different facets with different people.

In certain primate groups, for example, chimpanzee troops, females mate freely with all unrelated males. There isn't any fury or pecking order going on here—all the males still nurture and protect the female and her offspring, no matter who sired them. But in gorilla troops, the Alpha male has sole sexual control over all the females he desires—he'll actually assassinate the offspring of a previous Alpha male when he takes over, just to ensure his superiority. Pretty tough stuff. The multiple male–mating female troops are comfortable and tolerant; the restrictive Alpha male–dominated harem troops are violent and warlike. Which would you like to belong to?

Of course, we aren't about to convert to chimpanzee behavior in America today. Hardly anyone, even the most radical among us, are up for throwing out all the old rules without having some excellent guidelines for making new ones. There are a few—not too many—human cultures that have thrived on polygamy, where both multiple husbands and wives are permitted, but we don't live close to any of them, in body or in spirit. And so we keep our traditional partnerships—marriage or living in a monogamous relationship—to reduce jealousy and rage in society, to establish boundaries for child rearing and community development. And to keep ourselves sane.

Unfortunately, this system makes for big gaps in pleasure and in self-assertion. It leaves us prey to the opinions of others and tells us we are "bad" if we want something more from our sexuality than a stable base for our relationships.

Sex can be fun, a time out of time to throw off your clothes on a warm spring day and get sticky with sap as you roll around under a tree, laughing hysterically. It can also be intensely spiritual when you feel that you have left your body and become part of something much bigger than the two of you consummating a physical act. Love can alter the course of a life. It can hold people together over time and space, and even if they never see each other or speak on the phone, it's still there.

Sex and love can be split apart, and unlike Siamese twins joined at the head, they will not perish.

What Do You Think About Sex Outside Your Marriage?

The statistics on extracurricular sexual activity in America are elusive—*The New York Times* reported in 1993 that half of all married men have had affairs (with men or women) and more than a third of married women have had affairs (with men or women). Reader polls of various women's magazines report the figure at about 40 percent for women and 50 percent for men, though some recent sexologists gauge the figure at only 15 percent. Perhaps the variable numbers relate to the fact that no one is comfortable telling the truth about whether they do or don't.

If you make a decision today to be sexual with someone other than the person you consider your mate, you have a lot of thinking to do. By taking that step into another bedroom, you implicate more than yourself and your lover—you must consider your primary partner and your lover's primary partner. It's not only the issue of safer sex (see Chapter Five), but the innate danger to the order you've established in your world.

Affairs are distracting and unsettling and involve some element of lying (or omitting the complete truth) to those you love. They are difficult to manage if you don't have a discreet space in which to be together. And if this is in fact just an affair and you intend to stay with your primary partners, you are risking everything if you are discovered.

All these warnings may not deter you if you have your reasons for the affair in order, as Alice did. She had never contemplated sleeping with anyone other than her husband. And she had known the man who became her lover for three years before they ever touched.

She was the head chef in his family-owned restaurant and spent most of every afternoon and evening with Steve, his mother, and his three grown sons. His wife had died of cancer about five years earlier and he had a girlfriend he was serious about marrying. Alice was very much in love with the man she'd married sixteen years earlier—there was nothing out of place sexually or any other way with their marriage. Still, she found herself powerfully drawn to Steve in a way she couldn't explain.

"I was totally intrigued by him," Alice said. "I'd watch his body in the mirrors around the restaurant when I was on my breaks, and sometimes I'd see him look up and make eye contact with me. I blushed every time, like I was sixteen instead of forty-eight.

"Then one Sunday morning, I realized I'd left my glasses at work and I drove over to get them. Steve's van was in the lot. We went and sat out on the outdoor patio and he poured me a cup of coffee and gave me that look. I knew I was blushing and I started laughing.

.   "'What?' he asked.

"I just blurted it out, 'You know I've got a crush on you.'

He nodded, and then said, 'And I've got a crush on you. I guess we have to wait until our next life to do anything about it.'

"But a week after that, he kissed me in the walk-in refrigerator. A week after that, we made out in his van in the parking lot after everyone had gone home. And a month later, we went to a motel. Both of us kept saying, 'We're crazy, this can't be happening. It's not love, so what is it?' Two middle-aged people acting like kids.

"As to what I felt about my husband, well, I didn't feel at all guilty. I couldn't call what I was doing adultery or cheating or any of those labels society puts on an extramarital affair. My relationship with Steve was so separate from that with my husband, who's my true partner. There was never any question of my leaving my marriage. But I did find that the affair made me value my privacy, my own independent joy, my sense of exploration. The sex with each man was totally different, although they were both wonderful, and I grew more orgasmic with each of them after I started the affair.

"My attitude about marriage and fidelity changed radically. I don't think it's possible to be everything to just one person for your entire adult life. And I don't think monogamy necessarily guarantees marital fidelity, either. There are plenty of people who only sleep with their husband but don't really give themselves to the marriage, but stand outside it, pretending it's all perfect."

Others I interviewed for this book who had had affairs, like Alice, did not do so because there was anything substantially wrong with their marriages. They had been in mature, partnered relationships that included lots of good sex, yet they had met someone else who brought out a completely different side of their personality and allowed them to express their sexuality in a way they never thought possible before. This phenomenon is particularly true for individuals at midlife, when they are questioning all those "roads not traveled."

And there are other, more traditional reasons for affairs. If you have been in a sexually cold marriage for a long time, and your partner is either turned off to sex or is too ill to participate in a sexual relationship, you may begin to feel deprived of simple human physical contact. If your partner is abusive, physically, verbally or emotionally, you may find yourself unable to enjoy sex with this person.

Take apart the facets of you that desire sex and those that desire love. Then see if the affair is really worth the danger, the anxiety, the precautions you must take. You are justified in having a desire for many varieties of sexual contact; however, the problems you may face in pursuing them can be mammoth.

There's a final *caveat* to an affair: One or both of you may fall in love. Is it possible to be in love with your spouse and in love with your lover? Sure, it is. Understand how difficult it might be to end this kind of relationship.

Only you can figure out whether having a sexual relationship with a person other than your partner makes sense. The truth of the matter is, sex is *never* simple or uncomplicated, and you may find unwanted wrinkles appearing in the previously smooth fabric of your own thoughts about your sexuality. This is a hard choice, and only you know whether you are capable of making it.

Changing Your Expectations: From Sex to Sexuality

Changing your attitudes and approaches to your sexuality means going back to the very beginning, at the point when you first realized you were sexual. Those who study childhood development say that we are sexual from our first year of life, but it's only when we *realize* that we are sexual that we gain the power I'm describing. Some people are terrified by that realization and put the power in a drawer forever. Some are intrigued by it, but don't know how to use it. Some go with it, but are too hung up on how it affects their partners instead of themselves. Some experiment with so many varieties of it that it becomes meaningless busywork. There are those who are seriously dedicated to improving their sexual communication and achieve this higher level of sexuality after a long time, when the body itself is no longer in its physical prime, but the mind has developed in many interesting new directions.

Sexuality is bigger than you think—certainly much bigger than your sex life. By opening up the idea that you can use your attractiveness, creativity, and interpersonal imagination outside the bedroom, you will find that you begin to approach others very differently.

Eric, who performs a type of therapeutic bodywork called *kiatsu* told me that his friends always called on him when they had any aches or pains. "I love doing it," he said. "I feel so connected to the person I'm with—male or female—it's like I'm inside them. And I'm giving them relief of pain and a way to get their body back on track."

Margaret said she had a very sexual approach to her sensual work, although it didn't involve touch at all. As an interior designer, she is turned on by the idea of creating beauty around her clients. "They receive from me, and I give to them and then it switches. When the relationship is really clicking, we know that we're into something that's almost physical." Deep intensity with another person need not lead to the sex act; yet it may be sexual. You will have to play with your expectations and grow along with them. You will also have to be honest and direct with your partners who may not be up to your level of participation in this brave new world.

This is a responsibility, but it will be well worth your while to take it. By listening to the many voices of your sexuality—the joy, the pathos, the silliness—you can turn the improvisatory nature of a really wonderful sexual encounter into a better team effort at the office, a revitalized class full of eager students, or even a symphony.

Shake Up Your Mind—And Your Body

We will never reach a higher level of sexual awareness if we don't change our attitudes first. We have to rub out those first ideas about intimacy, the ones that came from the hushed tones and stifled whispers we heard as children. And these are so hard to erase!

We tend to hide sex, to do it in the dark, to think about it in stolen moments when no one else can intrude on our sometimes disturbing fantasies. Most of us are conditioned to keep sex under wraps—for some of us that heightens its allure; for others, it makes suspect the very enjoyment we get from it.

Some people use sex to cure what ails them for the moment: loneliness, anger, boredom, a feeling that you're not good enough can all be temporarily wiped out by the plunge into hot, thoughtless sex. But does this cure or just stick a Band-Aid on the hurt? It's kind of like eating a fast-food meal that tastes really good while you wolf it down, but half an hour later leaves you slightly queasy and wondering why you risked the calories and fat for a quick fix. Until we demystify sex, we will tramp through life with the same albatross we have carried for years, and never really be certain about our own needs and how to fulfill them.

Making Time, Feeling Secure

When you begin your personal journey into the *whys* of your new sexuality and an elimination of the *shoulds* of your old sexual attitudes, you will find that you need two very important elements.

It takes time to make love. To get in touch with your sexuality and share it with a partner, you have to spin it out for a few hours every so often. This way you can explore leisurely what you want, what you like, and how you can relate that to your partner's needs. A quickie, although fun every once in a while, will only satisfy your immediate sexual needs. The value of time will become enormously clear if you take an evening to talk together, touch each other (not exclusively on the genitals), do a variety of intimate activities together, like bathing or massage, and finally end up on the floor or in a bed making love. You need *time* to make this a whole body and mind experience (see Chapter Eleven, How to Make Love).

You also need security. You have to feel completely safe with another person to whom you have entrusted your body, emotions, and your unique method of balancing the power and energy between you. If you think you'll be laughed at, or you imagine that the other person is out to get you in some way—either physically threatening or humiliating you for his or her own purposes—you can never really relax. (And you probably shouldn't.) If you don't feel secure in the arms of another, this may be the wrong other and sex is undoubtedly the last thing you two should attempt.

Your sexuality grows as you grow, and like a mountain, the changes come slowly, over decades. But only if you give yourself the option of lots of time and lots of comfort.

A Little Laughter Goes a Long Way in Bed

When you're truly embarrassed because your foot got stuck in your underwear when you were trying to be oh so cool slipping out of them casually, laugh.

When you hear yourself making all sorts of noises that don't quite tabulate as human because you're so excited, accept it as appreciation when your partner laughs.

If you have an erection and lose it on the way to that precious opening, it's okay for both of you to laugh. Really.

Sex is funny. Think about this: the human body, with all its various curves and knobs and parts that move and parts that try to move but don't always achieve their goal, rubbing and thrusting and licking another person with the same curves and knobs in order to feel good.

Laughing in bed is one way of sharing intimacy, and people do it far too infrequently. The impetus to find sex amusing is a deeper part of the connection you have with someone else—this is a joke the two of you share, and no one else is allowed in the clubhouse. Laughter is forgiving, and it sets aside lumpy bodies and strange smells and hairs out of place or missing. It allows all forms of touch and expands the senses. It makes a place for the two of you in the universe. And it makes the whole thing fun, instead of deadly serious.

When you can laugh with another about all your foibles, you can heal those terrible perfectionist tendencies we all have—to look oh so sophisticated and sexy, to be everything to our partner, to give and receive pleasure in just the right amounts and the right ways. There isn't any right, and as soon as you accept yourself and your partner, warts and all, you are on the road to being a whole sexual person.

So laugh out loud, and let your partner do the same. You'll be sexual much more of the time out of bed because you'll both remember—and appreciate—the punch line.

QUIZ
Are You the Sexual Person You Want to Be?

The object of this test is to find the aspects of yourself that you are hiding, neglecting, or overusing. Your score will not tell you how "normal" you are; rather, it will point the way toward how much self-confidence you have about reaching your goals or setting new ones.

A score of 17 to 26 yesses means you're in touch with and acting on your desires; a score of 10 to 16 means you have some work to do on self-esteem and sexual goal setting; anything below ten means you are seriously hiding from yourself and would do well to open up a bit more, painful though it might be at first.

1. Do you have as much sex in your life as you'd like?

2. Do you initiate sex most of the time?

3. Do you engage in sexual activity only when your partner wants you to?

4. Do you always ensure your safety and your partner's by using a variety of protective sexual methods (contraception and barrier protection)?

5. If you are a heterosexual, have you ever acted on a desire to have a homosexual experience? If you are a homosexual, have you ever acted on a desire to have a heterosexual experience?

6. Do you frequently change the time and place where you make love?

7. Have you ever made love outside?

8. Have you ever made love in a semipublic area (movie theater, beach, parking lot)?

9. Have you ever spent a day in the nude?

10. Have you told your partner that you masturbate?

11. Have you masturbated in front of your partner?

12. Have you shared any of your fantasies with your partner?

13. Have you experimented with the feel of different textures (velvet, silk, linen, rubber, leather) in your sex play?

14. Within the past year, have you asked your partner to engage in an activity that neither of you have ever done?

15. Do you avoid engaging in sexual activity to get rid of other feelings, like anger or depression?

16. Do you flirt or become extremely personal with people when you want them to know your sexual intentions?

17. Do you avoid flirting or acting sexual with people you don't intend to follow through with?

18. Have you told your partner that there are certain things that don't please you in bed and you'd like to curtail them?

19. Do you reinforce the particular things you're crazy about in bed by actually telling your partner that you love them and would like more of them?

20. Do you talk about sex with your kids?

FOR MEN

21. If you can't get an erection, or lose your erection, will you continue being sexual in other ways despite this?

FOR WOMEN

22. If you are not sufficiently aroused to have an orgasm, are you honest if your partner asks whether you've come?

23. If you have a chronic physical condition, such as heart disease, osteoporosis, arthritis, or cancer, are you still enjoying a relatively active sex life?

24. If you are taking a medication that affects your sexual desire or performance, have you discussed changing your dosage or prescription with your physician?

25. Can you see yourself as a sexual person at age eighty or ninety?

26. If you could never have sex again, with yourself or another person, what would you substitute for the feelings you get about sexual excitement and release?

Sex in the dark is a learned behavior; sex in the sunlight can be liberating and enthralling. But we have to trust ourselves and our partners enough to look at one another—see the delicate hairs on a cheek, the rough surface of an elbow, the swell of the breast and nipple, the tumescence of the penis. To be even braver, we have to look one another in the eye and declare, "Yes, *this* is what I want!" And by changing your beliefs, you may discover that you have what you always longed for and never had the courage to claim as your own.

Safer,
Smarter,
Hotter Sex

*W*hen my generation plowed its way through our early adult years, we were blind to the potential hazards of sex. We could get pregnant or we could get the clap, but those could both be fixed without a lot of *sturm und drang*.

It's a whole new ball game out there. There are so many health risks involved in the sexual act, it is difficult to separate our longing for closeness from our hot-headed desire to take risks. There is, to start and finish with, the human immunodeficiency virus (HIV). And there are many other sexually transmitted diseases (STDs) that can get you. Along with disease and a shortened lifespan, there are emotional byproducts of not taking care of yourself and your partner.

So urgently, I ask you to protect yourself and anyone you sleep with. I don't want you to look at sexual behavior with a partner as a potential battleground. I want you to see it as a mammoth, ground-shaking event, one that involves physical and emotional care and responsibility on the part of you and your partner.

If you think of wearing condoms as protecting yourself from a dread disease, you color the nature of your relationship with mistrust and fear. If, on the other hand, you look at your decision to use condoms as a loving way of taking care of your partner, you add intimacy and consideration to the bond between you. Once you've learned to do that, the boundaries open up like blooming hibiscus, and limitations fall away.

*H*ow to Talk About Safer Sex with Your Partner

Most people never make sexual decisions. They simply allow passion to sweep them up for a brief time or allow lack of passion to guide them away from intimate encounters.

But these days, we not only have to make the decisions, we have to talk about them before we ever get near a bed. If we are car-

84

ing sexual beings, we have to think and rethink what we do with and for one another.

You have to talk about condoms. And I don't mean the brands and sizes and textures. You have to figure out together what using condoms means to you. A lot of people—usually women, but men as well—tell me they're embarrassed to carry condoms because maybe it implies that they're loose, or looking to get laid. Maybe it sends a message saying, "Honey, *I'm* in charge," that could be threatening to certain partners. Or maybe they don't want to confront the perennial complaint, "I can't feel a thing with rubbers on."

It takes a kind of skill to keep your own beliefs and convince another person to abide by them without seeming nasty, aggressive or cold. It takes practice to hang onto your self-esteem when someone's nibbling at your ear and whispering that they're so hot they can't wait and just this once without protection won't hurt.

It could hurt—a lot. Safer sex is not an option—it is a new way of life, and should be for everyone in our society, whether they are infected or not. So you must learn to say the words and convey the message effectively and compassionately. Practice makes it a little easier each time.

What to Say

Be honest if you care about each other, even if it's embarrassing to say what's on your mind. This is essential for really good sexual communication. Of course, you want to be tactful so as not to hurt your partner's feelings, but you must look the issue right in the face. Here are some of the things you might want to say to one another:

"We've run out of condoms, and I'm too much into being alone with you to run out to the drugstore. How about we just give each other a massage and do other fun things tonight. We could always have intercourse tomorrow."

"Here are the flavored condoms and dams so you can go down on me—God, do I love that!—and here's the regular latex with spermicide if we have intercourse."

"I love being with you, but I can't get hot if I don't feel comfortable. We need to use condoms."

Maybe the words sound silly or overly cautious. You can modulate what's being said with your tone of voice and the implied feeling behind your words. The more often you talk like this, the easier it will get. One elemental principle of honesty in sexual discussion is for each person to have a say, and for both of you to do as much—or more—listening than talking. Encourage your partners—if they're shy—to say what's on their minds.

You might recall one encounter when something wonderful, or terrible, happened and compare notes on it. You might share fantasies—explaining what you've always imagined doing but never had the guts to try. Talking about wild sexual practices doesn't mean you have to do them. But the excitement generated by telling one another things that turn you on can be catching, and inspiring.

---

*S*AFER SEX GUIDELINES

The Institute for Advanced Study of Human Sexuality has a sliding scale for sexual activity:

SAFE SEX PRACTICES

1. Sexual fantasies
2. Sex talk (romantic or erotic)
3. Flirting
4. Hugging
5. Dry kissing—any part of the body
6. Phone sex
7. Bathing together
8. Massage (nongenital)
9. Frottage (body rubbing, clothes on or off)
10. Smelling each others' bodies and body fluids
11. Licking (only on healthy, clean skin)
12. Masturbation (mutual or solitary)
13. Exhibitionism with mutual consent (watching your partner stimulate him or herself)
14. Stimulation to orgasm on any external body part (armpits, breasts, elbows, knees, feet) using a condom or latex dam

15. Using your own sex toys on yourselves, not sharing
16. Watching sex movies or tapes together
17. Reading erotic books or magazines together

SLIGHTLY RISKY SEX

1. French kissing
2. Stimulation to orgasm between thighs or buttocks (no penetration) with condom
3. Fellatio without ejaculation
4. Fellatio with ejaculation into a condom
5. Cunnilingus with a latex dam barrier
6. Anilingus with a latex dam barrier (rimming)
7. Digital–anal sex with glove or finger cot
8. Digital–anal sex without barrier
9. Vaginal intercourse with condom and spermicide
10. Anal intercourse with condom and spermicide
11. Contact with urine (golden showers or water sports on unbroken skin)

UNSAFE SEX

1. Vaginal intercourse without condom
2. Anal intercourse without condom
3. Swallowing semen
4. Swallowing menstrual blood
5. Swallowing vaginal fluids
6. Unprotected oral–anal contact (rimming)
7. Unprotected manual–anal intercourse (fisting)
8. Unprotected manual–vaginal intercourse
9. Sharing needles (although this is not a sexual activity, very often drugs are used to enhance sex).

Safer Sex for You and Your Partner

If you really want to be safe and you want to be sexual, it will be easier if you get rid of your old, outdated ideas about masturbation. Although this activity has always had an unsavory reputation, and many people harbor the old myth from childhood that masturbation is bad for you, self-stimulation when you're alone or in the presence of a partner can in fact be a very pleasurable experience. You can learn (and so can your partner, if he or she watches you masturbate) just what turns you on and figure out ways to prolong and hasten sexual excitement. You have ultimate control over your own body when you masturbate and therefore have unlimited potential to create a sexual experience that offers comfort, pleasure, and self-knowledge.

Masturbation in front of a partner and abstinence are the only two methods of completely "safe" sex between two people. When it comes to "*safer* sex," there's a great big palette of colors to choose from.

Use Your Imagination for Greater Pleasure

Think of how lovely it can be to remove one article of clothing after another from your partner. Unwrapping this big present and being rewarded with the sight and feel of skin. From there, stick with the outside of the body only. Massage, rubbing skin on skin, stimulating sexual organs with dry parts of the body (your penis under your partner's armpit, for example) or dry kissing are delightful and carry very limited risk.

Safer sex never has to be dull. Experiment, be creative. You can use different textures—a scarf, a piece of velvet, a leather belt—in your sex play. You can use a variety of helpful aids such as oils, bubble baths, ice cubes, and different kinds of food to share with one another or rub on one another and then lick off.

You can make the paraphernalia of sex into something funny or erotic or both. Condoms and dams can offer opportunities for rich and imaginative sex play. Practice putting a condom on your partner with your mouth—there's a challenge. Stretch the dam over different areas of the body and stick your tongue into different covered orifices, like the navel or the anus. There's hundreds of different methods of sexual stimulation—if only you have the exploratory ingenuity to discover it.

Protection Is Always Essential

Now once we leave the body's surface and delve within, we are not quite so safe. Every type of sex that involves penetration into a body orifice or cavity, if not protected, is risky. Although there are no documented cases of passing the HIV virus during cunnilingus or fellatio, the possibility certainly exists. Particularly if one of you has cuts in the mouth or gum area, or if one partner is a menstruating woman, oral sex can take place only after you have put a *latex dam* over the genital area and kept it in place during each and every encounter.

Unprotected genital and anal sex are the most problematic activities for transmission of any sexually transmitted disease. The mucous membranes of both areas are prime entry points for the virus through exchange of semen, precum, and vaginal or cervical fluid. The anus bears a double risk because it is less elastic than the vagina, and there is more chance of tearing the tiny blood vessels that surround the anal opening. If you do indulge in this type of sexual behavior, you can pass both blood and semen. There is also more friction involved in penetrating a tighter body area, which means that your condom is more likely to break during anal than vaginal or oral sex. Protection is vital if you're going to penetrate either the anus or vagina.

If you are both men, it is a wise idea to wear *two latex condoms and use nonoxynol-9 spermicide* from start to finish; if you are a man and a woman, the man should wear condoms and the woman may wish to further protect herself with a *diaphragm coated with nonoxynol-9*. There are also female condoms and specially constructed latex panties, available at some sex shops and through some HIV/AIDS clinics. If you're using condoms that already have spermicide in and around them, these have an expiration date—so you must check to see that your condom is timely before you use it.

If you find that you're allergic to the spermicide, or that it completely numbs the areas you had hoped to stimulate, there is an alternative. The Institute for Advanced Study of Human Sexuality markets a product called Erogel, which is *nonoxynol-15* and does not have the numbing or allergy-producing chemicals of nonoxynol-9. You can contact them at the address listed in the back of this book for more information.

As for other forms of protection, the sponge has *not* been found to be an effective barrier against the HIV virus or other STDs. All other forms of contraceptive—the pill, the IUD, and the cervical cap—will only help to prevent pregnancy and offer no protection against any virus.

$\mathcal{H}$ow to Have Fun and Stay Healthy with Condoms

It is time that sexually awake and aware men and women all got savvy about latex condoms, the ones in the packages specifically labeled "disease prevention." No animal skin condoms allowed—even if you think they feel better. They're too porous to keep out those microscopic viruses.

But latex works. Condoms made of this superior substance come in all sizes and shapes, lubricated and non-, smooth and ridged, with and without reservoirs in the tip to catch the ejaculate. They even come in colors and flavors, but beware of these—novelty condoms are attractive and fun but are only useful for oral contact—they aren't any safer than naked skin for vaginal or anal penetration. You'll have to put on a regular "disease prevention" condom afterwards if you want to perform penetrating acts.

Mix and match condoms. Buy lots and keep them everywhere—by your bedside, in the car, or wherever you may be having sex. Condoms have to be cool (don't keep them in your wallet or in the medicine cabinet beside a radiator). If they seem brittle or sticky when you take them from the package, throw them out! A rotten condom is as bad as none at all.

Condoms, even two at a time, are not safe without spermicide to kill viruses. Many brands of condoms come already coated with nonoxynol-9, and you can buy tubes of the stuff over the counter as well. If you or your partner likes it slick and slippery, add a water-based lubricant, particularly if your skin is very sensitive. Some of the brands you can use are KY Jelly, Replens, or Astroglide. Never use oil-based lubricants such as petroleum jelly, mineral oil, Crisco, or cold cream.

Treat condoms gently. Don't pull them or stretch them before use. If you've been condom-free most of your life, practice unrolling them when you're not in the throes of a sexual encounter. You can practice on yourself if you're a man, or use a banana or cucumber if you're a woman.

Here's how to put one on: Wait until you or your partner are completely erect. Remove the condom from the foil and unroll it about half an inch. This is the time to apply the spermicide if the condom doesn't contain it. If you're using a brand with a reservoir tip to catch the semen, pinch it a little to let the air out. If you have a condom without a tip, place it on the head of the penis and hold back about half an inch to create your own reservoir tip. (If your penis is uncircumcised, pull the foreskin back before putting the condom on.)

Unroll the condom all the way—it must cover the penis entirely. Now you can apply more spermicide and a water-based lubricant. Remember that in the heat of passion, with a great deal of friction and movement, a latex condom is susceptible to breaking. Latex is a form of rubber, but it's not made like the tough variety that goes into automobile tires. It's "soft-cured," to keep it comfortable and elastic on the penis, which gives it a certain fragility. The lubricant can keep it moist and soft, and also may prevent irritation—and this is important because a penis with an abrasion or skin lesion would be more likely to transmit an STD or the HIV virus.

Your partner can help you unroll the condom on your penis—as you get used to doing this together, you may discover all kinds of erotic play involved. (You may not want to include oral play with a spermicide-treated condom—it's not known what amount of nonoxynol-9 is safe to ingest.) Since the condom will be rather slippery at this point, you may have to hold onto the rim when penetration happens.

If the condom breaks or tears, stop! Get a new one. If it won't unroll all the way up the shaft of the penis to the scrotum, it's either defective or you haven't put it on properly. Get a new one. It can be suicidal to be stingy about condoms.

The next part, you know. Just have fun. Then, after ejaculation, don't wait for the penis to become flaccid. If you do, fluids can leak out the sides of the condom and into your partner. While the penis is still partly erect, grasp the rim of the condom again and withdraw slowly. Pull the condom gently off the penis and throw it in a plastic trash bag. Don't flush it down the toilet—it may float to the top of the tank or, if it does flush down, it can jam up sewers.

Then wash up. Take a shower together and enjoy the luxurious feeling of flesh on flesh. (If you're doing any penetrative action, you need another condom.) If you haven't got time for a shower, just wash your hands and genitals with soap and hot water.

Other Safe Sex Devices and How to Use Them

Mucous membranes are everywhere—the mouth and back of the throat are lined with them. If you're going to have oral sex, you still need protection. Although it is true that the stomach acids would probably kill the HIV virus if you ingested semen or vaginal fluid, it's the passageway down that can cause problems. So a latex dam barrier is essential if you're going to have oral sex with a woman or anilingus with a man or a woman.

A dam is a stretched-out piece of latex usually cut into 6- by 6-inch squares. It should be placed over the area you're going to lick or suck and kept there throughout the act. Like a condom, a dam is thin and fragile and can easily rip or tear. It should not be reused.

Dams are available from sex shops in colors and flavors and plain from dental supply companies—sometimes they sell them in rolls or sheets you can cut to size yourself. The easier dam, though, is a homemade one. Just cut a rolled condom up the center and then smooth it out flat for a similar-sized piece of latex (use the unlubricated brands for oral sex). You can also take a latex glove, cut off the four fingers, then cut up one side and have a bigger sheet of latex, with the thumb left to put your tongue in so you can do delicious things to your partner. Since many unlubricated condoms are coated with cornstarch, you may want to wipe them down with a damp towel before you begin oral sex. You can also add flavors of your own, but be sure to use foods that have no fats or oils in them that would destroy the latex. (See Chapter Eleven for a complete list.)

Gloves and finger cots are available at most pharmacies and should be used for manual stimulation. You never know when you or your partner may have minuscule cuts or abrasions on your hands, so covering up is always a good idea, particularly if you're going to insert a finger or fist into an orifice of the body.

There's a new condom for women you might want to try, although my feeling is that the Reality condom is an incredible turnoff—difficult to figure out, unaesthestic to use, and it takes so much cooperation that any two partners who are able to use it successfully are probably so much in sync they're mutually monogamous and don't need condoms anymore.

But for the record: This large, heavily lubricated sheath that lines the vagina comes in a pack of three for $7.50. It's made of strong polyurethane—twice as strong as latex—and is incredibly durable. There's about a 0.2 percent chance of breakage as opposed to 3 to 5 percent with a male condom. The end of this sheath is inserted like a diaphragm inside the vagina, tucked around the cervix. It is *very* slippery because of all the water-based lubricant in and around it, and it tends to pop out a lot until you've mastered the technique of insertion. When properly in place, the sheath hangs down like a plastic baggie outside the body to protect the labia, and the erect penis goes inside the baggie. If you're going to have oral sex with your female partner, by all means, have it before you put this device on!

The Truth About Sexually Transmitted Diseases

Sexually transmitted disease is a fact of life. It's been around as long as sex has been around. The STDs that used to be the major threats, syphilis and gonorrhea, have now taken a backseat to HIV, the viral epidemic that rages internationally and for which there is no cure. Other STDs such as pelvic inflammatory disease (PID) and chlamydia, the fastest-growing sexual disease in the United States, may not be fatal but can, in fact, permanently impair sexual and reproductive health if not caught and treated early on. Or better yet, prevented, with proper use of condoms and spermicide.

HIV

HIV is transmitted through sexual fluids, blood, and blood products. Researchers have been chasing this elusive creature for definitive answers for nearly fifteen years, with little success. No one understands it. No one can cure it.

HIV can be passed from partner to partner on one contact, or an infected person can sleep with fifty infected people and not pick it up. It can lie dormant in the body for five to twelve years undetected, slowly sapping the function of the immune system and allowing other opportunistic infections to take hold. Women now compose the fastest-growing segment of our population infected with the HIV virus.

I do not care about the credentials, lineage, gender, age, or orientation of the person you've decided to become intimate with. Everyone in the world is now in a high-risk group when it comes to transmitting the HIV virus during the sexual act. Don't tell me you're a college student and only had one partner; don't bother protesting that you're a widow of sixty who only slept with her husband. Anyone you sleep with can transmit the virus to you and anyone you've ever slept with may have had a partner who transmitted the virus. This means that you and your partner *both* need protection.

Sex without condoms and spermicide is Russian roulette. Yes, you can have sex with an infected person and not catch a thing. But the next time you try unprotected sex, or the next, or the next, your chances increase of getting a sexually transmitted disease. Viruses are tricky buggers, and many mutate greatly from one host to the other. A particularly strong strain may overpower you though a weaker one failed. You just never know.

One of the biggest myths about the HIV virus is that it restricts itself to certain groups who practice certain acts, deemed unnatural by church, and often by state. But, as we know, the virus doesn't discriminate—it just wants a nice moist environment like the mucous membranes of an anus or vagina in which to proliferate. So men who have sex with men, women who have sex with women, and men and women who have sex with one another all have the potential to infect one another.

The sex act is not the culprit! How can we blame behavior? Instead we ought to go after the bigoted people who refuse to educate themselves about how this virus works and make them sit down and learn something useful, like how not to pass the virus themselves. It should be clear by now that safer sex affords you the possibility of developing a richer, more satisfying sex life; one that always regards a sexual partner as a partner in prevention.

Protection is essential, but if you forgot, or you rationalized, or you were just plain stupid, testing is a good idea. You will not necessarily know that this virus is in your body for a very long time.

The first signs that you are infected may show up a couple of weeks after the unprotected sex that transmitted the virus. You might feel flulike symptoms such as fatigue, swollen lymph glands, nausea, or night sweats. Then, no signs at all, for months or even years. Men sometimes find out they are HIV infected when they get Kaposi's sarcoma (a cancer of the blood vessels) or PCP (*Pneumocystis carinii* pneumonia). Women, on the other hand, may first find that they have a yeast infection that won't respond to over-the-counter treatment. They often find out that they are infected when they are diagnosed with pelvic inflammatory disease or cervical cancer.

Although early treatment with the antiretroviral drugs AZT, ddI, or ddC, and a new one, d4T, to be approved in 1995, can slow the growth of this virus, there is no cure. The only cure is prevention.

Chlamydia

This infection is much more common in teenagers than gonorrhea. The first signs may be vaginitis in women and urethritis in men. There may be some slight pain and a little discharge or no symptoms at all. Untreated, this infection can cause pelvic inflammatory disease (PID) in women; in men, it can cause an inflammation of the part of the testes that carry the sperm. In both these cases, infertility may be the result. It may also be passed from mother to child in utero. Testing is done by taking a culture; treatment is a few weeks of a strong antibiotic.

Gonorrhea

This is a bacterial infection, again, hard to track because there are often no symptoms. Men may experience painful urination and a yellowish discharge; women may have some vaginal or pelvic discomfort. If gonorrhea goes untreated in either sex, it can spread to the joints and the valves of the heart. It can also be passed from mother to child in utero and cause infant blindness. A bacterial culture can detect this organism; treatment is antibiotics or a shot of penicillin.

Herpes

Herpes simplex type 1 causes cold sores and blisters on the mouth. Herpes simplex type 2 causes genital and anal sores. The virus is passed by direct contact with the lesions; it can even be passed through hand contact, if the hands have touched the blisters. These blisters first appear two to twenty days after the sexual contact. They are small and filled with fluid, sensitive to the touch. Accompanying swollen lymph glands, fever, and achiness may make the sufferer think it's the flu. But be on guard, because once in the body, the virus has a permanent home. Some people have active episodes infrequently when they're under stress or their resistance is low; some never have another. However, sex when the virus is active is a big risk factor for cervical cancer in women. Since it can also be transferred in utero, there is a danger of herpes encephalitis, a lethal brain infection, in the newborn child.

Herpes becomes more severe in an HIV-infected individual, since the two viruses interact and support one another. Anyone with herpes should have an HIV antibody test.

You treat herpes by applying antiviral ointments and also by keeping the body in good physical condition so the immune system is primed and strong. Also, no invasive sex during active episodes is allowed.

Unfortunately, herpes doesn't always make itself so clearly visible. *Asymptomatic herpes* is a manifestation of this disease. The individual doesn't have blisters or obvious herpetic outbreaks, but is still exceptionally contagious. To be truly safe, if you have herpes, you should use some form of barrier protection at all times, since viral shedding is always possible, even during seemingly herpes-free periods.

HPV (Human Papilloma Virus) Genital or Venereal Warts

HPV's major symptom is highly contagious pink-red and soft or yellow-gray and hard pustules forming a cauliflower pattern around the genitals or anus. This virus itches and can become inflamed. If left untreated, in women, these pustules can cause a blockage of the vaginal opening. Treatment is by cauterization (burning) with an electrical probe or by freezing.

Some HPV viruses, however, are too small to be detected, or are hidden deep in the female genital tract. A Pap smear should reveal these, and sometimes, doctors will put a vinegar solution on the area—if warts are present, they will turn white.

Although this is not a big problem in most people, it can contribute to factors leading to cervical cancer if untreated.

Syphilis

This bacterial infection enters the bloodstream through a break in the skin of the uninfected partner, who comes into contact with the infected partner's lesions (chancres) or rash. The first stage of the disease manifests itself with these painless blisters or chancres; the second stage presents as a rash on the palms of the hands and soles of the feet. The third stage begins as the organism moves around the body and attacks many different organs—the heart, liver, nervous system, and brain. Treatment, which is antibiotic therapy or penicillin, with follow-up blood tests every three months, must take place in the first two stages; the third stage is lethal.

Candida Albicans, Vaginitis, Trichomonas

Vaginal infections that cause itching, burning, and discharge, sometimes pain with urination or intercourse, are the scourge of many women's lives. Men may present with a burning sensation in the penis and a red, spotty appearance to the scrotal area and genitalia. Candida is treated with a course of antibiotics and/or antibiotic creams. A vaginal infection that doesn't respond to treatment may be a symptom of HIV–infection.

Getting Rid of Barriers to Good Sex: Alcohol, Drugs, and Nicotine

You know it's not safe to be stoned or drunk when you drive; why should you think it's less lethal to have sex when you're not in your right mind? It is virtually impossible to talk and think clearly about sexual choices if one or both of you are under the influence of any mood-altering drug, be it alcohol, nicotine, prescription drugs, potent herbs, and even some over-the-counter medications. They may impair your judgment, release your libido, and affect balance and accuracy so that it may be difficult or impossible to put on or take off a condom or use a dam properly. When you're under the influence, it's also hard to decide whether the partner who currently has you panting with desire is really the right partner for you.

Alcohol

Alcohol is the most commonly used drug in America. A drink or two will certainly decrease inhibition and make most of us feel at ease, cheery, warm, and expressive. Women shown an erotic film after ingesting alcohol reported that they felt increased arousal, although the clinical findings showed that vaginal blood flow had decreased as blood alcohol levels increased. Because their blood vessels didn't engorge as they would in a sober person, it was harder to reach orgasm, and even when they did, the climax was less intense than when they'd had no alcohol. It is certainly true that too much alcohol will dampen the most ardent erection in a man. And the decrease in desire and orgasmic capacity is lower in men as well.

Nicotine

Nicotine is a powerfully addicting drug. As soon as it gets into the bloodstream, it begins to act on the central nervous system, stimulating a release of various neurotransmitters, which in turn, trigger an outpouring of stress hormones. The heart rate increases, and adrenalin surges through the system. The very nerve synapses of the body are affected by nicotine.

Many of the same hormonal and neural triggers are set off during sexual arousal, as you may remember from Chapter Two. But if these reactions have already been set in motion from cigarette smoking, you've shot your wad—there's hardly any stimulus left for a sexual reaction. Nicotine tends to keep people calm when they're under stress and stimulates them when they're bored or fatigued—neither of which is beneficial in a passionate embrace.

The toxic chemicals in the cigarette smoke itself make less oxygen available to the lungs, the heart, and the brain. Since sex involves a certain amount of exertion and exercise, it's more difficult to have a rollicking good time because you can't breathe well and your heart may be pounding dangerously fast. And, finally, if you didn't need more proof that this activity interferes with great sex, people who smoke smell awful, and this is clearly a deterrent when you're getting close up and personal.

Drugs—Recreational and Medicinal

Drugs come in many shapes, sizes, and dosages, and a huge number of them affect sexual desire and performance adversely. Some prescription medications used to treat depression, high blood pressure, and elevated cholesterol levels, and some contraceptive drugs can suppress libido, potency, or orgasmic ability. If you have to take these medications, and you can't get an erection or feel your libido has taken a permanent vacation, you should speak with your physician about lower dosages or even a change in the particular medication you're taking.

The recreational drugs most often associated with enhanced sexual experience are *marijuana* (not a drug, but a potent herb), and *cocaine*, derived from the leaves of the coca plant. Most people who smoke grass feel enormously relaxed and sensually alert. Every sensory organ, from the eyes to the taste buds to the sense of touch, is enhanced under the influence of marijuana. Unfortunately, however, since motor coordination is severely affected by grass, performance generally suffers.

Cocaine is a brain stimulant that offers an immediate high followed by a sudden low. The drug typically makes people cranky and restless. It speeds up reaction time and often induces a sense of paranoia. The restlessness may induce a violent episode of physical activity (running might do just as well as sex), but the anxiety created by the drug generally makes intimacy impossible.

There is, of course, the notion of an aphrodisiac effect—can a drug heighten the time you spend making love and the excitement you get from the experience? Certain drugs are known to increase your libido because they target the hypothalamus, that center of the limbic system responsible for our pleasure-seeking instincts. They stimulate the release of dopamine, a neurotransmitter that helps brain cells communicate with one another. *Poppers (amyl nitrate)* fit into this category. They cause an immediate rushing sensation in the brain and usually enhance the intensity of orgasm. But believe me when I tell you that this high can be lethal. Poppers are exceptionally dangerous, and have been linked to Kaposi's sarcoma, a cancer that often accompanies HIV disease. Possibly more than any other recreational drug, this one should be avoided at all times.

Other drugs and herbs have substances that act like estrogen and testosterone, the body's sex hormones (see Chapter Two). Testosterone, which men and women both produce, is the biggest libido-enhancer the body creates. *Yohimbine*, when taken in excessive doses, has been shown to have a positive effect on libido and erections, probably due to its testosterone-like qualities. A similar reputation is held by *ginseng*, which is a highly estrogenic plant. But because the mind is the number-one source of sexual arousal, taking any herb with a sexy reputation probably works only if you believe in its effect.

We all crave the ultimate mind–body experience and lots of us will do anything to get there. The promise of an altered state of consciousness draws us on toward eternity and gives us a glimpse of something larger than life, bigger than ourselves. In our search to know something of what's beyond our world and our perception, we will try anything to achieve ecstasy. And yet, this is exactly the effect that sexual experience, all by itself, without any helpers, can give us if we pursue it to its extremes of bliss (see Chapter Thirteen).

Staying Healthy, Staying Hot

If you look at sex as genital or oral or anal satisfaction, you are seeing only a tiny piece of the entire sexual map. The most potent sexual organ in the body is the mind, because imagination is what sparks desire. The second most potent organ is the skin, and luckily, the outside of the skin is a fairly strong barrier to infection when intact. And you don't need a condom for either of these body parts.

Once you get used to considering other ways of making love, the disappointment in not getting the brass ring (traditional orgasm reached during genital or anal intercourse) will fade away. There are highly sensitive individuals who feel we can train ourselves to lift the sexual desire we all experience from the sexual organs and channel that energy up to the brain, creating more excitement and more meaningful connection to a partner.

Go back and look at the list of low-risk sexual behaviors. Start with the challenge of simply exploring the body in new ways.

The sexual act is only a small part of your sexuality. People who care about each other tend to value their common interests, their coinciding senses of humor, their ability to communicate openly with one another, their tolerance for each other's quirks and habits, their ability to experience a range of emotions together—from fury to annoyance to comfort to love, and their acceptance for and admiration of the other's way of being. After all those qualities, after the intellectual and emotional attraction for the other, comes the importance of feeling physically attracted.

Hot sex is hot because of the way we perceive it, and this astounding facility will be with us until the day we die, if we're lucky.

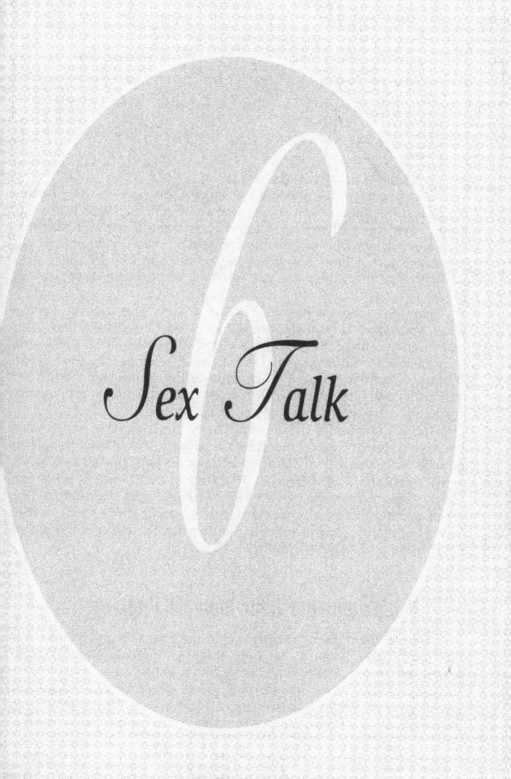

6

Sex Talk

"*I* want to make you come."

Nancy shivered, repeating her lover's sentence to me. "I can't tell you how this aroused me—I feel weak just saying it again out loud. When he told me he wanted to make me come, I was his. Those words showed me his singleminded desire to do something wonderful to me, like he wasn't going to stop until he got there. And it wasn't just the words, but the intensity in his voice. It set me on fire."

Um. Talk can be delicious. What a rush goes up your spine when your lover is saying these things to you! Your brain and body take them in, imagining what it's going to be like when the words turn to deeds. Nancy is turned on, as most of us are, by the verbalization of fantasy. She can imagine, standing across the room from her lover—everything that will happen between them, just by the suggestion implied in that one sentence. So simple.

Yet so difficult for most people. Why do we have so much trouble saying the words? As much as I've always encouraged people to go wild with words, I've stuttered and stammered myself asking for what I want. It's not so hard to do things in the dark, but when we speak the unspeakable, we're self-conscious about sounding like we're auditioning for a porno film. And so sex is often silent, sometimes boring, sometimes painful, sometimes lacking in any kind of oomph—just because no one will talk the talk.

Liberating Your Sexual Language

Words are certainly mightier than swords, so maybe the words for "penis" and "vagina" are even mightier than the organs themselves. When we're very little, we're told it's not polite to use "bathroom language." Don't talk dirty! Some of us were spanked just for knowing what certain words mean, and for others, that taste of soap in the mouth is a remembrance tantamount to Proust's *madeleine*.

104

Funny how this works out in adult life. *Doing* uninhibited physical acts in the midst of sexual passion is understandable, but freely
expressing ideas is not. "I wasn't myself," many people say after carrying on like a wild banshee, but what can they say after speaking
words that could be controlled or bit back if they just thought a little
more clearly?

Suppose you tell your lover about a fantasy that involves being
tied to the railroad tracks and being raped by three men. Will he
think you're nuts? Will he be worried that his performance in bed
could never measure up to what you have in your mind? People
often take fantasy as true expression of desire—which just isn't so in
most cases. We all have imaginations and can conjure up exceptionally bizarre circumstances that we find stimulating. This is perfectly
normal. But most of us don't act on the weirdest ones, nor do we
expect a partner to create that fantasy in real life for us.

So why talk about them? Because it's private, it's intimate and
it gives your lover yet another way of knowing you. It also opens the
door for some interesting ideas that maybe you haven't tried out yet.

Same goes double for discussion about what you like and don't
like during sex. If you can say what turns you on (and many people
really aren't sure, which is why I so strongly urge you to play with
each other and experiment), you can get more of it. Why is that such
a hard thing to ask for?

What stops you from talking honestly?

- worry about being censured by your partner for your thoughts
  and feelings, some of which may make you feel guilty or
  embarrassed.

- concern about intruding on your partner's privacy, and yet during a shared sex act, privacy becomes a two-person street, to
  be traveled jointly.

- anxiety about spoiling the mood, because you were brought up
  to believe that magical sex just happens between two people
  who are so in sync with each other they know instinctively,
  without being told, what to do.

- awkwardness about saying words you don't say in public.
  Unaccustomed as you are to using the language of sex, you will
  only become more comfortable if you practice. And the only
  place to do that is during a sexual encounter!

- lack of understanding of how your partner thinks, because he or she has problems talking, too. Deborah Tannen, the doyenne of male–female communication and author of *You Just Don't Understand*, explains that men and women actually perceive words and their meanings in different ways.

Express Yourself with Your Own Brand of Sex Talk

It isn't what you say so much as how you say it. The flavor of your language is part of your personality, part of your sexual appeal to a partner. Some people talk baby talk to a lover; some a foreign language they happen to share. Some will create a private means of communication based on shared experiences the two have had.

You have to get it out in the open if you want to heal old sexual hangups and start on the road to a healthier sex life. It's important to take that risk and speak out. You don't have to do it all at once; you can work your way into it gradually. And again, it will be helpful if you let your partner know what you're doing—and you have to talk about that, too!

How do you usually express yourself in an everyday situation? Once you've figured that out, you can better decide how you want to express yourself sexually. Are you a contemplative person who weighs the pros and cons before verbalizing one succinct thought? Are you a witty, clever master of repartee? Do you jump from one topic to another, seamlessly weaving them together to make your point? When you've pinpointed the type of talk that naturally emanates from you, you'll be better able to translate that when you want to communicate sexually.

How to Turn Each Other On Telephonically

Phone sex is a particularly wonderful way to spin out your most brilliant fantasies. No one can see you, so you feel perfectly safe and not quite as silly as if you were face to face with your lover. It's almost like being alone and reminding yourself of your hottest desires. Jared, an artist's rep, told me he called his girlfriend any time he knew they couldn't see each other for a few days. It drove the two of them crazy with lust.

"I said things I'd probably never say to her if she were there—I have no idea what came over me. Like I wanted her to get over to my office that afternoon wearing just her jean skirt and bolero jacket and heels—and no underpants. I wanted her to walk in like she was coming for an interview and hike up her skirt a little and sit on my leather love seat. Then I'd sit across the room and tell her to spread her bare legs and I'd explain in detail how I'd go down on her, but I wouldn't even have to touch her to see how wet she was already.

"It was the most incredible aphrodisiac for the two of us. We couldn't wait to get together. I think it kept all the juices flowing in our relationship, just thinking about what we'd do when we finally connected."

Phone sex is not only a great turn-on, it's safer than anything else two people can do together sexually. It's also wonderful practice for talking in bed, since the phone serves as something like a confessional. If you can't see or be seen by the other person, you tend to let go a little more. Learning to be erotic and honest telephonically can help with more advanced couple-talking, when you have some real problems to work out.

Getting to Know You, Sexually

How does anyone know what you like and don't like unless you tell them? But so few of us do! We like to think that the bonds of closeness between individuals are so mystical, they even cause interlocking brain waves.

"She should have known I'm incredibly sensitive, and it can hurt if she keeps fondling or sucking me after I come," said John, a forty-year-old contractor who'd been divorced twice and was now contemplating a third marriage. I asked how his girlfriend was supposed to know this, and he shrugged. I explained that unless he actually said something, she might assume that he was pushing her hand away because he was annoyed or fed up with her.

If it's really too hard to hear yourself speak the words, you can use shorthand: "more," "harder," "softer," and just plain, "yes," will do it.

After a sexual encounter, when you are thinking about what just happened between you, some people get really emotional and it comes out verbally. Alice, whom we met in Chapter Four, said that as she was going through menopause, she used to cry a lot after sex, but only with her husband, never her lover. She had to talk to him about why, although it was extremely personal—more so than the sex itself. "I said I wasn't crying from sadness but more at the thought that the time allotted to us was passing. There was such a rush of feeling between us after sex, and that was wonderful, but I knew that even if we had thirty or forty more years together, it was going to end. I never felt that with my lover, because our relationship was temporary, anyway. We were never going to chuck it all and run off to Tahiti together."

Other people find that after sex is a good time to "review" things that went on. If you let your lover know you really were crazy about the way she cradled your penis with her breasts, she'll remember to do it again sometime. If you say the words, "It's the best thing in the world when you slide in and out of me slowly like you did for the longest time tonight," your partner will have more than a clue as to what you really like in bed.

Go Ahead! Say "Dirty" Words

The dictionary is filled with hundreds of possibilities, and street slang gives you a whole different lexicon. Just listen to the sound of Latin words: "coi*tion*, masturba*tion*, fornica*tion*, flagella*tion*." If you'll pardon the pun, many think these activities, like the words that label them, should be shunned at all costs.

Using "dirty words" may be one way of breaking the accepted rules of polite society. If you can say it, you can sexualize it. This can be good practice for those who were taught that sex didn't exist without love and only love made the physical part all right. Lots of little girls were brought up to believe that the knight in white armor was an appropriate object of desire because he would sweep you off your feet without removing your clothes. So you couldn't tell him you were aching for him or that you longed to unzip his pants because it would make you too vulnerable, too open for rejection. And it would make your sexual nature too obvious, when you were trying to be mysterious about it.

Men don't usually have a problem talking dirty with other men but may avoid it with women whom they regard as too genteel and fragile to take all this heat. But if a man is able to tell a partner what drives him wild and what he wants to do, this may open the door for some badly needed communication. The dirty words can be a symbol of the gutsy, juicy nature of our sexuality. Maybe if we all loosened up, and talked the talk, we could make a dent in society's expectations.

What does it say about you if you find dirty words a turn-on? It may mean that you have no guilt about expressing your true sexual feelings. Name-calling may be a substitute for the real thing, though—some rather repressed people talk up a storm but are surprisingly uncreative in bed.

Remember, healthy sex is a time for adults to play with one another, and talking dirty is something we loved doing as kids, when our whole life was play. Then, too, when you're in the midst of a passionate encounter, and fireworks are exploding from all parts of you, including your vocal apparatus, you may not even be aware of what you're saying. Moans, grunts, screams, and every word you ever heard or read may pour out of you.

But what if your partner is grossed out by the slang you select? Although you may mean the sentence, "Your pussy is so hot," in a tender and loving way, your lover may feel you're being vulgar. People with lower self-esteem may also take the comment as a criticism because of the shock value of the word you use.

If you feel like talking dirty, don't hold back. It certainly can't hurt and may spice things up between you. But you must stay aware of your partner's reaction. If you sense a cringing or disapproval, you've got to discuss the matter together—preferably out of bed (see below).

Use Flattery to Work Wonders In and Out of Bed

Several people interviewed for this book said that what they most wanted to hear from a partner was flattery. Someone who tells you that you look better in short shorts than anyone else on the planet, or that you have the greatest, warmest mouth they've ever felt, or that, quite simply, you look fabulous, is on the right track verbally. Does you partner always mean the exaggeratedly wonderful things he or she says to you? It depends. Getting on your good side may be a way to persuade you to do things you didn't originally intend to do. But, on the other hand, flattery before, during, and after sex can be the most sincere statement of how much you mean to your partner.

The question comes up about the word "love" all the time. Some people, in the heat of the moment, tell a partner they love him or her. And because this word is so emotionally loaded, it can change the whole mood of your encounter. That one potent word can flatten an erection or squelch an orgasm. So talk about it! Love isn't the same thing to any of us; in fact, it isn't the same thing for any one of us from day to day or moment to moment. You may certainly have loving feelings toward a person you aren't in love with. But if the word makes your partner run in the opposite direction, it's not worth it. And if you are waiting around, eager and anxious to hear only that word from a partner, you may be barking up the wrong sexual tree.

Not all kind words are honest, but sometimes, they serve a purpose that goes beyond truth. As Bill, a social worker, described his first male lover's approach from the vantage point of being forty, he realized his college professor could never have thought he was so prodigiously smart as he indicated. "He encouraged my academic work, told me how incredibly brilliant I was and how my work stimulated him. He rewarded me with wonderful dinners and nights at the theater and opera and said that my being there made the performances so much more meaningful. It was such an adventure getting all this experience with him, all the while getting so appreciated just for enjoying the new stuff he was giving me. I didn't think of his praise as flattery, but now I see it for what it was. And it did get me into bed with him."

Take flattery as it's intended—part of the process of pleasuring a lover. Saying to someone, "You excite me every time I see you," is going to make them feel wonderful. And then, you really will be excited because your partner will feel a sense of accomplishment in what he or she is doing. As long as you aren't too greedy for compliments, flattery is a healthy way to enhance a sexual encounter.

*H*ow to Say What You Want Without Hurting Feelings

The gold standard of a good relationship is one where you can talk about anything. Not that every action and lack of action has to be chewed over together, but important issues have to come up. My husband and I had been together for almost fourteen years before we ever divulged the fact that we masturbated!

When you look at this closely, it makes sense. If you love someone, you can't bear the thought of hurting him. And although the sexual experience you have during masturbation is entirely different from the one you have with a partner, it still may bring up feelings of competition or rejection. If I tell him, will he think he's not "enough" for me? If he doesn't do the same thing himself, will he understand or be really turned off?

It's even more difficult to discuss things that we want the other person to do or not do. If we say it wrong, it can come out sounding like criticism.

So how do you say what you want to tactfully but truthfully? You can start by asking your partner's opinion about the activity you're interested in trying. "Have you ever known anyone who did X?" or "Did you hear about that couple who were into Y?" is a good way to open the channel. The next step is to confess that you're interested in, although maybe a little nervous about, doing it. And when you tell your partner that he or she is the only one you'd ever trust to try something this daring, you have flattery at work again.

What Shouldn't You Say?

My personal feeling is that some secrets are essential to our innate sense of wholeness and should not be shared.

Let us take, for example, thoughts that you think would be disturbing to a partner because you know that person well enough. You may have had homosexual fantasies that would be incredibly threatening to your mate. You may not even have any desire to act on them, but just discussing them could create a barrier between you. In this case, better not talk to your partner about it.

Let us take, next, an affair that you have had or are currently in the midst of. Many people experiment outside a marriage so that they can force an issue with their spouse—they *want* their mate to find out so that they can wreak havoc with the settled relationship they now think they have. The motivations for this type of behavior may be revenge, a power play, a sincere desire to shake up the marriage and make it work better—or a need to end the marriage.

But for people who have extracurricular affairs for other reasons, possibly because a spouse is chronically ill and incapable of sexual activity, telling could destroy the relationship. If you love your spouse and don't intend to let the affair influence the course of your marriage, keep quiet. And that goes for dear, close friends. It may be difficult to keep this information all to yourself, but it could be a terribly hurtful mistake to confide in someone who knows your spouse and might slip by word or deed. It's also an unfair responsibility with which to saddle a good friend. A therapist, on the other hand, is an obvious choice of confidant.

How to Talk Without Words: The Power of Nonverbal Cues

Jack, who is a never-married musician and meets a great many women through work, describes himself as a quiet person who doesn't use words casually. "I want a woman to be direct, to say what she really wants, and I do the same for her. But I can't stand the idea of sounding like an idiot. I would assume if I talked like that to somebody in bed, she'd laugh hysterically. That might not be bad, except it would break the mood. Dirty talk is like being overly observant in your chosen religion to my way of thinking—it's so ritualized and formal."

Jack talks about nonverbal cues that let him know something sexual is about to happen. "It's like a situation you're in which looks perfectly average, but has a separate meaning. I remember I invited this woman for Sunday brunch about a week after we'd met at a mutual friend's house. I was sitting at the end of the couch and she came and sat on the arm of it next to me, kind of in position to be kissed. Then there's eye contact—the first time we met, she looked at me and I couldn't look away. I was so turned on. Everything was heightened; that moment took on a life of its own."

There are a variety of nonverbal cues that let couples know that something is about to happen between them. If you aren't attuned to these, it's time to brush up your skills. Waiting and watching can be extremely stimulating, a prelude of what's to come. When you're quiet together, you are sharing something deeper than a superficial conversation.

But it's not always easy to interpret the meaning of that silence, particularly in the sexual realm. Even married couples have problems learning when one wants to and the other doesn't. When your partner adjourns to the bedroom at 9 P.M., is she asking you to come with her, or is she just tired? It's okay not to understand, especially if you haven't lived together that long. It doesn't make you insensitive or out of sync with your spouse's moods. When in doubt, ask (it's time to use some words)! If we don't check on situations like these, things can fester inside. These unspoken problems can lead to trouble in a relationship.

Nonverbal cues can easily be misinterpreted. Some people are just very "touchy," and what appears to be enormous personal interest in you may be their routine way of interacting with anyone and everyone. This can trigger jealousies in newly married couples. If you see your partner responding physically to others the same way she does to you, maybe it's time to talk about those messages you want to give and those you have no intention of sending out.

Then there is the problem of gift-giving and favor-doing. Some people will bend over backwards to get things for you if you casually mention that you want them. Is this an overture, or just a kindness?

If you always greet a friend with a peck on the lips and one day he starts opening his mouth on yours, is the next step an invitation to a secluded back room? When in doubt, ask! It is because we keep silent about situations like these that we get into terrible trouble with sexual harassment. Miscommunication between the sexes is a well-documented phenomenon. Men's and women's brains are actually wired differently, particularly in the areas that affect social interaction. When you accept a nonverbal cue without questioning or stopping it, you give back a nonverbal message that whatever's going on is okay. If you don't want to give that message, go back to square one and find out what the other person's real intention is.

Finally, there are the cues that need not be misinterpreted, but often are because most of us have been taught since earliest childhood that the human body has to be covered to be safe and sound. Those individuals who feel that a physician is making a pass when he asks that all clothing be removed during an office visit and then proceeds to do a thorough visual and tactile examination of the body need to reassess their values. Of course there are deviants in the medical profession as there are in any other field; however, it is not necessarily true that all doctors are perverts. They have to *see* the naked body to check for symmetry, alignment, lesions, rashes, discolorations, and so on. I find it curious that gynecologists (mostly male) routinely drape their female patients when they exam the genitalia; no internist or urologist (also mostly male) would do the same with a man having a prostate exam.

Don't be paranoid, certainly not around the person you love. You can be pretty safe if you take most nonverbal cues at face value. Sometimes, when a friend hands you a banana, it's just because he thinks you might be hungry.

How to Let Your Partner Know You Want To

Use your five senses as they were meant to be used: as powerful attractants and receivers of stimuli around you. In order to send erotic messages to your partner, you don't need a pad and pencil. Just open your mind to all the possibilities of your body's cues.

- The eyes are probably the greatest source of nonverbal communication. Just a look, or the way the look lingers, is important between couples. In your daily contact with friends and acquaintances, when you make intense eye contact, people look away because it's embarrassing. But in a love relationship, the gaze that rivets you to one another can be overwhelmingly intense. Some partners are so close, they describe being able to contact their beloved visually even when their back is turned. There's an energy that comes through the eyes, "the window to the soul," that pervades the loudest cocktail party.

- Look at the setting, examine the room, the lighting, the atmosphere. On the surface, everything may seem perfectly ordinary, but there may be a hidden meaning. For example, if you arrive at your lover's house in the middle of the day and all the shades are drawn, that could serve as a big neon sign blinking the message that your partner is interested in making love.

- Think about the position you get into when you want to be close. If you're sitting at the end of the couch and she avoids every other piece of furniture in the room in order to sit beside you, she is implying that she wants to get even closer than she is.

- You might move so that your bodies accidentally brush, and then not break the contact.
- You might place a hand on the shoulder or back of your loved one when you're talking about something totally innocuous. The quality of your touch might show that you have stopped whatever it is you've been doing just to appreciate the other person physically being there.
- You might hand your partner a glass and let your fingers linger on hers.
- You might lick or purse your lips in a significant way.
- You might smile, thinking of a private joke between you. Some couples can transmit the punchline without words.
- You might change the tone and quality of your voice.

All of these cues can provide a stimulus to lovemaking, and not a word need be spoken. Your whole body may respond to being turned on—your presence may seem bigger or warmer to a lover who is attuned to what's happening between you.

How to Listen and Talk Out of Bed

If the two of you are having problems in bed, don't let them drag on. They *will* get worse if you don't talk about them. There are many things that could go wrong between you, but they don't have to stay that way. Some lovers are tormented with conflicting amounts of desire (one is always ready for action and the other seems to simmer on a low flame). Some couples have serious or temporary sexual dysfunctions like painful sex or premature ejaculation. They may miss cues and suffer from a lack of good timing—which ends up with only one or neither partner being sufficiently pleasured by the experience.

It's not a good idea to take the erotic arena and turn it into a battleground. So if things are uncomfortable in bed, save your discussion for the next day. Make a lunch date to talk—this can be a cheese sandwich on the back porch, nothing fancy—just an opportunity to be alone together in a nonsexual setting.

Cars have been a popular place for conversations that must be private but shouldn't be anywhere near the area of conflict. (Of course, you run the risk of having an accident if the sexual tension between you escalates.)

It can be traumatic to sit down and analyze what's the matter—and it may take professional guidance. Several sessions with a counselor or sex therapist may be the best route to learning how to talk—and how to work on the problem.

What you say to one another may be halting, may sound dumb, but the fact that you've opened your hearts to work out what's wrong means that you're on the right track. Think before you say the words so that they mean what you want them to mean and are not hurtful.

QUIZ
How Big Is Your Sexual Vocabulary?

The point of this quiz is not only to test yourself on the number of terms and slang words you know, but also to find out how fluent you are in expressing your wants and needs. Try the answers on for size—several in each group may be correct.

1. If I tell you I love frottage, does it mean
   a. I am committed to safer sex?
   b. I enjoy using cheese as a sexual stimulant?
   c. I would like to rub your penis between my thighs or buttocks?
   d. I like to be spanked?

2. If I tell you I think Kegels are great, am I talking about
   a. a sex toy?
   b. an exercise for my pubococcygeal muscles?
   c. an additional stimulus to enhance orgasm?
   d. a new rock band?

3. Will you stop me from engaging in irrumation if you're worried about HIV transmission?
   a. not if we're wearing protection
   b. yes
   c. no
   d. only if I wear braces or one of us has cuts in our mouth

4. How should you ask me to stop doing an activity that you find less than exciting and start doing something else?

    a. "Oh, I loved that thing you were doing before with your tongue. Could you do that again?"

    b. "I just don't get turned on by that."

    c. "Cut that out."

    d. "You drive me crazy. Do you want to make me even more nuts about you? Let me tell you how . . ."

5. If I want you to go down on me, I could say,

    a. "Tongue me, sweetheart."

    b. "Eat me, please."

    c. "I love it when you put your mouth on me."

    d. A nonverbal cue of moving up in the bed or steering your partner's head in the right direction.

6. If I say I've practiced the act of intromission, does it mean

    a. I've had sex?

    b. I've cheated on my partner?

    c. I'm a lesbian?

    d. I'm celibate?

7. If I tell you I want to try infibulation, does it mean,

    a. I could be gay or straight?

    b. I'm into kinky sex?

    c. I'm at high risk for HIV transmission?

    d. I enjoy more than one sex partner at a time?

8. How could I tell you I enjoy cuddling after sex?

    a. "Stay with me, I'm lonely for you."

    b. "You look like you're about to leave."

    c. "Turn over. You must need a backrub after all that strenuous activity."

    d. "Don't fall asleep yet. Let me turn on some music and read you a section from this book that really reminds me of you."

9. How could I tell you I want to experiment more?

    a. "Let's not bore each other with that again."

b. "I have a great idea. What's your favorite food?"

c. "Have you ever done it in the bathtub?"

d. "This may sound crazy to you, but I'd love to make love to you in your office with the door locked."

10. If I say I'm interested in tribadism, does this mean.

a. I'm lesbian?

b. I use sex toys?

c. I want to do group sex?

d. I extend my sexuality into the realm of feminist statement?

ANSWERS:

1. a and c; frottage is French for "rubbing"

2. b and c; Kegels are exercises developed by a physician for women recovering from labor and delivery. They are also used in a program of training for incontinence and are enormously beneficial in sexual pleasuring, both yourself and a partner. Both men and women can do Kegels by squeezing the pubo-coccygeal muscles (muscles around the perineum).

3. a and d; irrumation is the act of moving the penis inside the mouth.

4. a and d.

5. all.

6. a. Intromission is the act of placing the penis into an orifice, either mouth, vagina or anus.

7. a, b, c, and maybe d. Infibulation is body piercing, usually with the intent of placing a ring or other ornament in the new opening. This can be a very dangerous practice because it leaves the body open to bleeding and infection.

8. c and d. Stating that you're lonely or that you perceive the other person isn't interested since the act itself is over is a real turn-off.

9. b, c, and d.

10. a, b, and maybe d. Tribadism is an activity between lesbian partners where one assumes the male role by strapping on a dildo and entering her partner with it.

7

Healing Your Sexual Self-image

*I*f you hate yourself—or any part of yourself—you can't show yourself off, you can't dance with abandon, and you can't joyfully surrender to another in bed. I am really sad and mad about the fact that many people truly believe that they must look "great" in order to be sexy. Where's the standard? Who made the mold we're supposed to conform to?

No one can give you definite parameters for looking "great" because there aren't any. You have unique appeal, as does your partner, as does everyone on this planet. The real trick is finding it and cherishing it.

How do you turn yourself on so as to reach out to others sexually? Are you actually brave enough to do that?

So many of us spend whole decades of life preoccupied with the way we look and how we appear to others. The media's immaculate brainwashing about our age, size, shape, smell, and configuration has brilliantly erased any semblance of good feelings many of us might have about the wondrous differences of the human form. But we can overthrow the mean-minded media and the nasty little creature who sits on our shoulder saying, "you're not gorgeous enough or macho enough to be sexy." The real sexual healing, however, works from the inside out.

*D*o You Like Yourself Enough to Be Sexual?

Ever heard yourself saying the following?
"My breasts are okay, but my butt is huge!"
"How can I go the beach if I don't lose five pounds?"
"I ate four pieces of pizza—I'm such a pig!"
"I've got a hundred things to do before I see Joe: shave my legs, tweeze my eyebrows, use mouthwash, put on perfume, and find that pair of black pants that camouflages my horrible hips."

"She's going to jump a mile when she smells my breath."

Why not do a hundred sit-ups before getting into bed? Or starve yourself for a week? Or have a face lift? Not so far-fetched, eh? Some do.

Men and women typically have their own personal nutsiness about their bodies. There are exceptions to all rules, of course, but most men interviewed for this book crave being larger in some way (penises, amount of hair on the head, and muscles lead the list). The only things they want to shrink are love handles.

But nearly every woman interviewed wants to be smaller.

The word "feminine" implies dainty and petite—therefore, with the exception of breast tissue, women find themselves craving a diminution of their hips, thighs, butts, stomachs, calves, and ankles. They hate deep wrinkles and large noses. (No one ever compares sizes of clitorises and labia, which is interesting, since every woman's are different. But since we aren't taught to look at ourselves "down there," we never get to the point of jealous comparisons.)

I recently heard a woman on a radio talk show about body image call to say that she *knew*, objectively, that she was very attractive. And this was her problem. She was so dependent on the idea of being perfect that she spent most of her time worrying about whether she really looked as good as she could at that particular time. She was unable to relate to others—male or female—because she was so bound up with her anxieties about her looks.

I asked each person I interviewed for this book what made them feel sexy, and some were at a complete loss for words. They had never thought of themselves as sexually attractive! Those who had the best self-images tended to pick something that was not a physical attribute you can work on in a gym, like pecs or butts. The most sexual people credited their eyes or their smile with their ability to go forward in the world like a magnet, making others zing irresistibly toward them.

Angela, now in her fifties, had been beaten into self-hatred by a set of horrifying circumstances that conspired to eradicate her sexual well-being. Sexually abused by her father, and unable to tell her mentally ill mother who'd been institutionalized, she confided in a priest. He determined that she'd "asked for it" and that she was to go home and "honor her father." She was gang-raped in sixth grade, pregnant at sixteen, and sent off by her furious father to a home for unwed mothers.

"Sex became something I had to have, like a cup of coffee, like going to sleep and waking up. I didn't connect it with any emotion, I was like an instrument to a man—he picked me up and played me."

Angela's self-image changed when she met a woman who really cared for her. "I went to a bar one night just to try it, to 'be gay,' and I met someone. I was never comfortable with the sex part of this, but I liked the fact that I never had chemistry problems with the woman I lived with. She cared for me, she showed me it was possible. After this relationship, I lost all the weight I'd been carrying. I'd been afraid of my attractiveness, and being thin made me feel vulnerable and unsure. But when I started to be okay with who I was, then getting thin showed that I could accomplish something."

Angela's husband, whom she met a year later, had a much more idealized notion of what they could be together. "He thought all the bad stuff would go away when we were married, and he went through hell when he found out love didn't conquer all. But I'll tell you, he did help me a lot because he changed my whole attitude about myself sexually. He made me see how I didn't have to be a victim, didn't have to be an object for someone else's pleasure. One thing I had with my husband was that hand-in-glove feeling—we just fit. It wasn't man and woman; inwardly, we had no gender, we were just humans."

He died in 1990, and Angela has been celibate since then, although she can foresee another relationship in her future. "People sexualize things too much—it's not your partner who turns you on, it's you. You liking you being with someone else."

How can you learn to like yourself? First, you must find out what you *don't* like. There are three basic roots of your self-image—your sexual, physical, and emotional selves.

Sexual Self	Physical Self	Emotional Self
Attractiveness	Attractiveness	Self-esteem
Fertility	Fertility	Assertiveness
Feelings for another	General health	Feelings for other
"Dirty" or "exciting"	Cleanliness	Independence
Gender identity	Ability to perform	Vulnerability

You can see that there's a lot of cross-over. What we consider "attractive" physically and sexually translates as our self-esteem emotionally. We may have old ingrained attitudes about sex being either "dirty" or "exciting," but on the other hand, we are still preoccupied with how we will smell to a lover if we've just come back from jogging or we have our period.

The bigger issue of sexual identity is orientation—which sex are we attracted to and why. And this question comes head-on with fears of being able to perform that cross the boundaries of heterosexuality or homosexuality. We are all vulnerable in front of a partner. This is what makes sex so scary and so fabulous at the same time.

There is another big issue here, which so many of us have to confront. If we were abused, as Angela and so many others were, if we were brought up to believe that everything about us was rotten to the core, how do we heal this? Even for those who haven't been sexually abused as children or as battered wives, many suffer from intense self-loathing because they don't measure up to the plastic values of Madison Avenue and Hollywood. Think how awful it would be to compare yourself daily to Wonderwoman or Superman and kick yourself about why you couldn't measure up sexually. The answer: because you were never supposed to.

It will take a sympathetic partner who is both sexually giving and verbally eloquent about just how wonderful you are to start to break down the destructive messages you've received over the years. For some, it may take some professional counseling. But the effort, believe me, is worth it. If you can like yourself on the street, in the office, in your child's playground, at a cocktail party, or anywhere else, you can like yourself in bed.

How to See Yourself as Others See You

When you are always looking at yourself through *your* version of *someone else's* opinion, you are bound to be wrong. You're so critical! So picky! If you walk onto a beach and are certain that every person there is riveted on your cellulite or your flabby arms or your hairy back, you are giving yourself an awful lot of credit.

The fact is that most people are busy thinking about themselves—unless they are really involved with you, they don't give you much thinking space at all. This is hard for some people to hear,

because their ego demands that everyone pay attention, even if it's
a rotten kind of attention.

EXERCISE
Introduce Subtle Changes to Your Image

Try the following:

1. Change something subtle about yourself and see if your partner
   notices. (Two unmatched socks, belt worn back to front.)
2. The first day of the week, dress exactly as you think your partner would like you to dress; the next day, dress as you would
   like to. Repeat over the next two days, then see what it is that
   makes the clothing different. Check with your partner to compare and contrast.
3. In bed, consciously do something to pleasure your partner;
   then ask for something you'd like your partner to do for you.

When you can perform these exercises thinking for yourself,
doing exactly what you want, you will have reached a milestone in
your self-esteem boosting.

How to Wipe Out Self-Criticism for Good

Do you think that other people are looking at you, judging you?
About how long do you think this has been going on? We saw in
Chapter Four that our notions of our sexual selves started forming
very early. We were looked at and cuddled or shoved away by a parent who was all-powerful. If you were rejected, you learned to take
it and move on. If you were accepted, you beamed with pride and
grew shinier each day. If you don't think your parents' opinions influenced you much, stop and look at them, and then at your siblings,
for a clue to the feelings you have about yourself.

In our first year of life, our "self-image" isn't formed—we actually see ourselves as an extension of our mother. As we grow to tod-
dlerhood, we separate and begin to form an image of who we are,

relative to our parents. This early separation is a preview of what's to come in adolescence, when we make a real break with home and family and strike out for our independence by sounding, looking, acting, and being different from our parents.

And at the same time, think of the transformation that's going on in our body image. No longer can we rely on the childish form that reacted in predictable ways and made us feel safe and sound. Suddenly voices crack, breasts stick out, pimples sprout—we can't cover ourselves up in the ideal child body anymore. We don't even recognize ourselves in the mirror. And we may hate what we see, particularly as we compare ourselves to others (of course, they hate what *they* see, too, but that's no comfort because we can't believe it).

As we get older, we are shaped by the world around us, and those we choose to let into our circle. A woman who sets herself up with abusive partners is stuck in a victim mentality. This abuse can take the form of criticism of the way she looks or behaves, and the longer it goes on, the more difficult it is to correct the imbalance of poor self-image.

Marsha, whose parents dominated her completely, had struggled all her life to speak up and express her opinions. Her sexuality was on hold, she thought, until she could make herself attractive to her husband. She couldn't even approach him, because her feelings about herself centered on his disapproval of her—how she looked, the sound of her voice, the way she related to his parents. (She was never able to see that his avoidance of her sexually probably had to do with deep-seated problems of his own.)

Every time she had a breakthrough, and told him what she thought or started a new project she was particularly proud of, he'd either ridicule it or ignore her totally. When she finally felt ready to initiate a romantic evening, and touched him, clearly opening herself for an embrace, he walked across the room and turned on the television. It was not until she was able to get herself out from the burden of this marriage that she could change her approach to life and take credit for doing it *for herself and no one else.*

Some people don't need a partner to criticize them. Something in their lives—being born without a limb, going through disfiguring surgery, or living with chronic illness, for example, can change the way people see themselves sexually. We'll discuss these perceptions later in the chapter.

Dare to Be Vulnerable with Your Partner

The thing about sex is that you usually take off your clothes. And, then, someone else has to look at you naked. This is something we don't do in any other context in life, other than bathing or sleeping, in which case we have to assume that we know the other person pretty well anyway.

QUIZ
What Are Your Feelings About Your Body?

Ask yourself the following questions and answer with brutal honesty:

1. When I undress, do I do it all at once or in pieces?

2. Do I keep the area I'm ashamed of covered until the last possible moment?

3. Do I make moves to camouflage the parts of myself that cause me to feel fearful and exposed?

4. Do I help my partner undress? Watch passively? Turn away so that I don't see?

5. Am I more likely to turn away from my lover's embrace if I'm menstruating and fear that I might not smell or taste desirable? If I'm ill or injured and feel less attractive?

6. Are there times when it's harder for me to undress? If I've just gained a few pounds or if I haven't been working out?

7. Are there times when I enjoy undressing for my lover—when I've lost weight or have made progress in an exercise regimen, for example?

8. Are there ever times when I'm not self-conscious at all about the way I look, act, smell, or taste? When?

9. Do I enjoy making love with the lights on?

10. What parts of myself and my lover do I look at when I'm making love?

How revealing this quiz is! When you think about yourself naked, it's almost more difficult than *being* naked. When we can give up the shame of the idea of showing another person exactly what we look like, who we are, and what we desire, only then can we be healthy sexual individuals.

EXERCISE
Reverse Your Getting-Naked Patterns

If you are currently partnered, go back through the quiz questions and purposely reverse some of the ways you typically respond. Your partner will be the best barometer of the way you feel about yourself. Remember, the idea is not to act in the way you think your partner wants you to, but to open your hand and show all your cards. You need a sympathetic partner who will reverse roles with you and expose his or her own vulnerabilities. Doing this exercise will allow you to be vulnerable together and will help to establish a strong connection between you. By giving up the things you've held onto (secrets, fears, anxieties), you will deliver feelings along with your body to the person you trust.

Talk to Your Partner About Yourself

Because the way you see yourself is such a pivotal issue in sexuality, and so personal, it's essential to check with someone else about your self-image.

Celia had battled her weight for years, and had finally discovered in her thirties that she liked being a big person. Her lover had wanted her for many reasons that were not physical, but he was definitely turned on by her size. He was also sensitive enough to her long-term battle with image to tell her that what he loved about her was her skin. He would rub his hands over her round belly, proclaiming it the most beautiful part of her. It was always the part she had hated the most.

He would never have known how to express this excitement to her, however, if she hadn't confessed her fears to him. At first she was only able to do this nonverbally, shyly pushing his hands away or trying to pull in her stomach muscles. Finally, when he asked why he couldn't touch her there, she admitted that she despised her fat belly. He was so surprised (because this was his favorite part) that thereafter, he made a point of emphasizing his pleasure.

A sensitive problem can be alleviated by a skillful exchange. It's a you-show-me-yours, I'll-show-you-mine idea. Just as expressing your fantasies to a partner can enliven your sex life (see Chapter Ten), so getting to the heart of your anxiety can vastly improve things between you.

When you are able to say what you don't like about yourself, your partner may respond with his or her own personal hang-ups. Neither of you will be able to wipe out years of self-hatred; you will, however, be able to acknowledge instead of deny reasons that you may turn away, turn off, or be unable to have an orgasm.

Change What You Can, Accept What You Can't

You will never achieve your personal ideal of beauty. Sorry, but you won't. You have been conditioned over the years to expect people to respond to a cardboard cut-out of beauty and handsomeness. What we see on television and in magazines is just a convenient shorthand that stands for a real human form, invested with all its natural grace and majesty.

In reality, there's a range of attractiveness that goes way beyond media images. The person who thinks you are hot stuff likes you the way you are. And you are not simply a sum of your parts.

Suppose you are vaulting toward menopause and have been having hot flashes periodically throughout the day. Do you really think it's unattractive to sweat on a date? If you believe that you're supposed to look fresh and "ladylike," you will be incredibly self-conscious about flashing. Instead, try to widen your perspective on the situation.

Everyone sweats. If you'd made a date to go running instead of have dinner, you both would have been wet most of the time. If your relationship eventually leads to the bedroom, you will soon find that you are getting moist in a variety of places. So no sweat!

Suppose your hairline is receding and you've become terribly self-conscious about your encroaching baldness. You are unable to imagine yourself as Sean Connery, who, without hair, is one of the most attractive men in the world. If you begin to comb your strands in odd patterns across your head, you are fooling no one but yourself. If, on the other hand, you keep what's left neatly trimmed and wear your scalp proudly, your self-confidence will shine through and make you more attractive. It has been said that some women are incredibly turned on by a bare head, which reminds them of a different type of head, also bare.

Believe me—you are the only one who notices your glistening upper lip, the pimple on your nose, or your five additional pounds. And none of them are important sexually.

Recovery of Self-image After Surgery

If you woke up tomorrow without your arms, how would you feel? Angry at your loss, puzzled as to why it happened to you, and incredibly self-conscious about looking different from everyone else. Although people would get used to your new appearance, you would always know that somehow you were defective, you were missing something.

That's exactly the feeling of a person who has had a breast or some internal organ removed or some natural biological function taken away that was given at birth.

How do you heal from these wounds? When you take off your clothes in front of the mirror, and then, in front of your lover, what can you do to feel whole again?

MASTECTOMY. A woman's two breasts define her to the world from puberty as female. They are the ultimate giving and receiving organs, they sustain new life, they sit in perfect synchrony, a set of heavenly hills rising from the flat plain of the torso.

After a single or double mastectomy, a woman must realign her thinking about her body and her attractiveness to a potential partner. Edith, a woman in her late seventies, told me that she had a new boyfriend and they were close to being intimate. She had had both breasts surgically removed over twenty years earlier, one had been reconstructed using tissue from her belly and the other had a saline implant. "Every time he starts to touch me when we're kissing, I kind of yank him around to the side. I think he's very confused. I feel like I have this awful secret and I want to tell, but I could lose everything. I guess, though, it's worse to me than it could be to him, because he didn't know me with real breasts before. I've started spending some time looking at myself in a mirror, and I discovered they weren't so bad. Maybe, soon, I'll be able to show him."

Some couples can't face the nudity issue right away, and this is perfectly fine. You can use lingerie, scarves, and other cover-ups to veil yourself erotically like Scheherazade.

Postsurgery, you will probably experience

- tenderness at the site; if you've had radical surgery where lymph nodes have been removed, also pain and difficulty lifting the arm
- fatigue
- anxiety about looking at the wound
- anxiety about touching or being touched there
- discomfort with nudity

Although about a quarter of women who've had this disfiguring surgery are depressed and anxious afterward, the real difference in sexual interest and excitement is in the group who receive chemotherapy. The debilitating effect of the toxic chemicals on the body can cause the ovaries to stop functioning, which is tantamount to an immediate menopause. Vaginal dryness, lack of libido, vulvar soreness, and a burning pain with intercourse are common. Nausea, hair loss, and weight loss contribute to your feeling ill and undesirable. The side-effects of chemo can be handled with medication and lubricants. Be sure you tell your partner which times of day you're least exhausted and just how much activity you're ready for.

The way you adjust to your sexuality after mastectomy depends greatly on whether you have loved feeling sexual in the past. If sex was never very important to you, or you saw it as an obligation, you may use your surgery as a reason to avoid intimacy. If, however, you crave the experience of touching and being touched sexually, you will find a way back to it eventually. Be patient, because it will take time. You will probably need some form of counseling, alone and with your partner if you have one, to recoup and restructure your sex life. The more support you have, the faster you'll heal.

COLOSTOMY, ILEOSTOMY. Since the days of our toilet training, most of us have had a horror of touching, smelling, or being close to our waste. Though bathroom functions are as routine as tooth brushing or bathing, the idea of combining sex and toileting is abhorrent to most.

But it's a fact of life. If you can no longer pass fecal matter through your bowel because of certain illnesses or pathology, you'll have it surgically rerouted. And for you, that will become the normal state of affairs. You can adjust what you do sexually as soon as you get over your old attitudes about the way it "should" be.

When an opening is made into the abdominal cavity from the small intestine (ileostomy) or the colon (colostomy), either temporarily so that a wound site can heal properly, or permanently, you must wear a bag to collect the feces. But a good nurse practitioner, who approaches ostomy care in a nonthreatening, compassionate way, can make it easier for both partners to adjust.

Clean the stoma site before sex, and empty the bag, if it's a reusable one; change it if it's not. In the case of a sigmoid colostomy, you may need only a gauze pad covering.

There is nothing else you have to know physically—the bag can be moved aside during sex, and waste collection should not be a problem if you have a good nutritionist who's explained in detail about your diet. Some ostomy patients can set a schedule for their elimination by changing the nature of what they eat. You can control odors, gas, and irritation by eliminating foods such as cabbage, cauliflower, broccoli, green beans, nuts, and seeds.

The embarrassment and emotional hang-ups about sex with an ostomy can cause a good many readjustment problems, but together, you and your partner can reach a comfort level that works for both of you. You will both have to get used to seeing and touching an area of the body in a slightly different way—but remember, your ostomy hasn't made you less sexual; only your inhibitions would do that if you let them. Follow the guidelines for mastectomy recovery given earlier.

HYSTERECTOMY. If it is absolutely necessary for you to lose your uterus, it can be a life-saving procedure. Unfortunately, this too common operation wreaks havoc with many women's self-image, because this organ signifies the core of our femininity. And although it's hidden (unlike a breast), so nobody need know that it's gone, it has enormously emotional power and significance in our lives. Although there are women who are relieved to be rid of periods and concerns about contraception, most tend to feel the loss of their uterus acutely, whether or not they've borne children.

The good news is that in a routine hysterectomy, only the uterus and cervix are removed. Because your vagina remains intact, there's no difference in your ability to have intercourse, and because the ovaries are still in place, there's no change in hormonal output.

The more radical procedure, an *oophorectomy*, where the ovaries and often all the reproductive organs (uterus, cervix and Fallopian tubes) are removed, causes an immediate surgical menopause. This can bring with it a variety of symptoms, such as vaginal dryness and hot flashes.

For about six weeks after surgery, you won't be able to do any lifting or heavy labor. You undoubtedly won't feel very sexual for several weeks—but then, you might not after any major surgery.

Even though sex isn't supposed to feel any different, many women emphatically affirm that it does. A decline in libido may occur because of a decrease in the circulating androgens—and these are the hormones that make us feel sexy. Also, if your mind tells you that you feel less feminine, your hormones would undoubtedly react to these powerful brain signals. Estrogen replacement therapy, often with a testosterone component to it, can replace sexual awareness and interest. But only a woman who is willing to delve deeper into her desires and fears, and a partner who can take that journey with her, will heal successfully.

VASECTOMY OR PROSTATE SURGERY. Every man has probably fantasized once or twice about repopulating the world with all his billions of potent sperm. After a vasectomy—the male method of permanent contraception—this dream is dashed. The operation itself is a simple procedure, but what an emotional punch it packs.

Under local anesthesia, a small cut is made on each side of the scrotum to reveal the two tubes of the vas which ordinarily carries the sperm from the seminal vesicles and the prostate. The tubes are cut and cauterized, then put back inside the scrotal sac, which is closed with a dissolving stitch. A relatively new procedure known as a microvasectomy is less invasive, requiring only a one-eighth-inch puncture to extract the vas. There is less time involved, less pain, less possibility of infection.

Don't think you can change your mind about this one. Although some physicians claim they can reverse the procedure and restore male fertility by splicing the cauterized ends of the tubes, in most cases, this isn't possible. You'll have to come to terms with a lot of heavy feelings about robbing the "family jewels" and about killing off all potential offspring in one's line. Even the least paternal of the male gender get the heebee-jeebees about this (as if it weren't bad enough having someone apply a scalpel to their private parts).

Recuperation involves wearing an athletic support and packing the swollen, sore scrotum in ice for about a day. Tylenol (not aspirin, which promotes bleeding) will generally alleviate the physical pain. A man is not technically sterile for the next six weeks while the vas clears, so a condom should be worn during this time to prevent pregnancy—and you still have to keep wearing them if you aren't in a mutually monogamous relationship (see Chapter Five on safer sex).

The psychological pain of "shooting blanks" may require some time—and a sympathetic partner. Many men want to prove that they're still manly and may feel an obsessive need to have lots of sex after surgery (wait about two days, at least). Since no alteration has been made to the penis during this procedure, there's no reason to fear that erection problems would result.

After prostate or testicular surgery, men will have a dry orgasm without ejaculation since they can no longer produce semen. It may be difficult to achieve an erection as well, but in men under the age of sixty, this can reverse itself in about six months. In Chapter Nine, I'll talk about the ramifications of physical aids. But a man will have many similar feelings losing a testicle as a woman does losing a breast. And though there's no hormonal basis for a change in sexual desire, it may take several months to recuperate emotionally from this type of surgery.

REMINDERS.

- After any surgery that involves the sex organs, you will have to come back slowly to yourself and to your partner.

- Talk to each other about your fears and desires.

- Masturbate (if so inclined), so that you can relearn what you need to know about your own pleasure.

- Use sensate focus exercises (see Chapter Eleven) to learn how to get excited all over again.

- Use water-based lubricants after any female surgery to increase sensitivity and make penetration easier.

Celebrating What Gives You Pleasure About Yourself

It is time for all of us to stop beating ourselves up for whatever shortcomings we think we have. We have been criticized by parents, teachers, friends, lovers, but most strictly and cruelly by ourselves. We agonize over whether we measure up at play as well as at work, and most of us are so competitive, we cannot look in a mirror without seeing another (better, prettier, stronger, sexier) individual standing right beside us, jeering.

If you are a prime offender in the self-denigration arena, it is time to pat yourself on the back (or some other body part). Your immediate reaction to the exercises I suggest below will probably be that they're not working. All the more reason to keep going until you see a difference in your self-image. It can happen if you believe in yourself.

How to Feel Better About Yourself

1. GO OUT OR STAY IN AND EXERCISE. More than anything else, more than a face lift, a new set of clothes, a new car or a new diet, *physical exercise* can make a huge difference in your sex life. Studies have shown that even those people who hate their bodies feel so much better about themselves after entering a program of regular exercise that they may be better able to deal with showing themselves naked to a partner.

Regular exercise really will enhance your sex life—men who entered aerobic programs and were monitored for sexual behavior were more willing to try out different positions and activities, they found that their erections were more reliable and they enjoyed more satisfying orgasms. I have to put a caveat on this—*too* much exercise reduces fertility—ultramarathoners have lowered testosterone levels, and women who exercise fanatically may lose ovarian function.

Exercise does make everyone feel better, however. There are so many benefits, from the toning of the skin and musculature to the deep breathing which gets more oxygen flowing to the brain, to the accelerated blood flow, the stimulation of the nervous system and the release of endorphins, the body's natural opiates that alleviate pain. What happens when we exercise regularly is that we are able to create a neurophysiological state similar to the one experienced by mystics and meditators. This allow us to feel better about everything in the universe, including ourselves and our partner.

2. SELF-APPRECIATION EXERCISES.

- *Past/present systems check.* Compare the you of today with the callow you who used to be. You may find that parts of your body and personality that were unformed have really come into focus for you lately. Then, too, the more mature you are, the more experience you have, the more self-confident you can be with a lover. You've been here longer, and therefore you know more. Congratulate yourself on growing up!

- *Giving yourself positive feedback.* The following exercise will allow you to understand that we are all unique and there is something wonderful in you that no one else can claim.

  Spend some time alone each day appreciating yourself. You might start with something easy that you've always admired about yourself. Maybe you have great eyelashes or terrific feet. Make sure you tell yourself why you like this facet of yourself. Add another part of your body or mind each week, but don't forget to go back to the ones you've already included.

  It may seem strange to establish your self-esteem on something as flimsy as an eyelash, but learning to stop and admire the least and most of life can teach you a lot about yourself.

You can heal yourself sexually by growing to enjoy and forgive yourself. Remember, whether you currently have a partner or not, you are a sexual being with your own unique beauty and fascination. The depths of your potential lie within your ability to cherish your individual quirks: the way you run a fingernail along your cheek, the way you shrug, the warmth in your eyes, the way you approach another person who may be hurt or depressed.

Give yourself credit. Lots of it.

Your Sexual Clock

*I*t starts ticking as early as the first year of life, and, if we're lucky, continues until death. Sexual interest and ability grow as we grow, so we have an unlimited potential to hone our sexuality over the years and let it color other areas of our life.

Time moves us forward. As our own seasons change, our inclinations and desires change as well.

*D*aily, Monthly, and Seasonal Fluctuations of Desire

We are different sexual beings at different times in our life—either ignoring our sexuality or reveling in it in adolescence and young adulthood, taking it for granted or working on it diligently during our adult years, mourning it or experimenting with it during midlife, cherishing it or forgetting about it entirely during our later years.

Some of us, who are particularly attuned to our sexual proclivities and interests, can actually chart monthly, weekly, and daily fluctuations of desire and activity. One woman interviewed for this book said that around menopause, her sexuality had begun to change daily—she related differently to herself and to others in radically shifting ways. It was exhilarating and self-revealing. "It wasn't that I felt sexy or didn't," Alice said, "it was more that the parts of me that were sexual had relevance to different aspects of my life at different times."

Since our sexual feelings have a great deal to do with the perceptions we get from our nerve endings about touch and pressure

138

and temperature, we can say that one person's pain is another's pleasure. Some of us are aroused by being hot; some by being cold. Some individuals are turned on in the winter, but most are sexier in summer. Several people interviewed for this book said they were always tanner and thinner in summer and felt better in their bodies, so sex felt better, too. But others loved watching the snow fall and cuddling; still others thought the very best sex was out in the brisk fall weather on top of a pile of jewel-colored leaves.

Most mammals cycle according to temperature and light conditions so as to bring forth their young in the good weather when there's plenty of food around—there aren't any wild kittens born between October and February for this reason. A female fox will wait until February to act "foxy." She attracts and mates with a male of her choice during her estrus cycle and remains with her mate after the birth of the pups and throughout the summer. Male deer, whose sexual proclivities have been extensively studied, have higher testosterone levels in late summer and fall when their antlers grow in. Thus the probable derivation of the word, "horny." Most mammals who carry their young for at least half a year bear them in the spring. Humans, due to contraception and planned parenting, have messed around with this neat pattern.

Some individuals love being sexual in daylight, possibly because their eye's stimulus is soothed by light and they may be depressed or frightened by darkness. The reverse is true of others who find the glare of light less mysterious and romantic than their desire dictates.

And there's a hormonal trigger as well: men's testosterone levels are highest in the morning, falling by late afternoon. At night, the levels rise again. The time of year is also important—American men tend to have higher testosterone from April to October than during the rest of the year. Women's monthly estrogen and progesterone production don't specifically affect desire and arousal. Like men, their androgens are responsible for libido, and these remain more constant in women throughout the days, the months, and the seasons.

Of course, there are many additional factors that let us know when it's the perfect time to come together sexually. The life cycle in both sexes is the biggest sexual clock we've got. Let's take it apart to see how it alters our sexuality over the years.

Your Sexual Timeline

The brilliant thing about human evolution is that we all start as mewling, helpless creatures and grow in a relatively short period of time into powerful, capable adults. Our sexual prowess grows as our body matures, and if we pay attention to our physical changes, we can augment them in many ways.

Infancy and Childhood

As infants and toddlers, we exult in the sense of touch. We thrive from the touch of a mother's or father's hands on us, the touch of the breast as we suckle, the touch, a little later, of our own genitals which allows us to differentiate ourselves as separate beings from our parents.

These infant genitals are small, but willing. Luckily, the almost ubiquitous male preoccupation with the size of the penis doesn't begin at birth, because baby boys have a half-inch to one-inch penis—which can become erect—and small testicles in the scrotal sac. About three percent of all newborn males and 30 percent of premature newborns have one or two undescended testicles. About half of these come down by themselves during the first two months and about 80 percent descend during the first year. Parents tend to panic about this condition, but most pediatric urologists take a wait-and-see attitude. Some doctors will actually wait until puberty for surgery. This is a hard call, since the emotional trauma of having that area cut at this age may be overwhelming.

Now we look at the tiny female genitalia. Baby girls have a small vaginal opening behind their urethra and in front of their anus. Girls can lubricate even at this impressionable age, and, like boy babies, have orgasms.

As we grow and become verbal, we can examine and name the parts and functions of our bodies. What toddler isn't delighted to discover the great world that lies between his or her legs during the toilet-training process? Penises and vaginas are the best toys, and children are usually fascinated with their form and function. They generally find out at this stage that they can give themselves great pleasure by stimulating their sexual organs—and if their parents aren't alarmed, they'll grow up to respect and enjoy the wonderful feeling of masturbation. As long as a child knows that this is a strictly private activity, there's no reason why he or she shouldn't indulge.

During the preschool years, playing doctor is in. Kids can help their friends of both genders on the road to sexual knowledge by exploring anatomy and reveling in their physical similarities and differences.

During the ages of five to about eight or nine, there is less obvious interest in the genitals, although many school-age children masturbate to comfort themselves. There are no significant changes in the reproductive organs during this time, except, of course, that they grow along with the rest of the child.

Preadolescence

And then comes the revolution, the time of heightened excitement, raging hormones, and a demand for the independence to explore this brave new world. Adolescence in America today begins at about ages ten to twelve. (The age for the onset of menses in girls and for testicular enlargement in boys has gotten progressively younger over the last fifty years.)

Girls have their first period anywhere from age nine to age sixteen; their ovaries, uterus, and vagina grow larger, and breasts begin to bud. They are self-conscious about their new bodies and alternately hate and love them. (Some teenage girls hate their bodies so much and crave perfection so deeply, they starve themselves into a grotesque version of the feminine. Bulimia and anorexia are not solely the province of girls, but boys tend to handle their fears in different kinds of self-destructive behavior, such as alcohol and drug abuse.) If you recall this time in your own life, you know that it is both highly stimulating and terribly embarrassing.

While girls can be humiliated by their upstanding breasts and unpredictable periods, boys of about eleven or twelve are crowing with pride over the growth of both their testicles and penis, which attain their final size at around age fourteen or fifteen. A boy knows he has become a man when he has his first nocturnal emission, the spontaneous ejaculation of various hormonal secretions during sleep. This usually happens about a year after his penis has enlarged. About this time, the pubic hair grows in and, as vocal chords lengthen, boys' voices croak and break. On the way down to a comfortable baritone, each boy has nightmares that he will be stuck forever as an alto-soprano. And all because of testosterone!

But it is also thanks to this grand gonadal hormone that a boy starts feeling his strength—he would never develop his potential male muscle mass if he didn't have the necessary adolescent increase in testosterone production.

The physical and emotional changes of puberty open the door to the scary world of adulthood. These extraordinary differences can give a preteen the feeling of the werewolf changing under the influence of the moon. There's no control over what's going on in your body—it just happens—and you are transformed whether you want to be or not.

Adolescence

What is this dramatic change good for, with all its agonies and frustrations? The survival of the species, of course. If we didn't get those brimming breasts and pulsing penises in our teen years, we might never go on to mate and conceive another generation.

You can probably remember feeling like the first person in the world ever to be attracted to a member of your own sex, or the opposite sex. You were the first to wake up sticky and soaked when you had your first ejaculation; you were the first to stain your white dress because you just never could count on when your period was coming. And who are you, anyway? Child, adult, male, female, loner, or part of a group? The identity crisis we typically experience during adolescence is part of becoming an independent, self-sufficient individual.

To deal with the fears and confusion, many teens become rampantly sexual. Their overt acting out has to do with testing, of course, and covering up for feelings of inadequacy. Many people I interviewed for this book said that their first kiss or "make-out session," which invariably took place at summer camp or some other setting where adults were not so much in evidence, was not pleasant. Men told me of the shame of trying to get close to a girl who rejected or laughed at them; women recounted stories about feeling forced to perform or give in. Usually the first kiss was not with a person that they enjoyed spending time with or were particularly attracted to. It was, rather, a rite of passage, getting rid of one form of awkwardness so that you could pass onto the next. (Masturbation, on the other hand, seemed to cause less anxiety. Most of the people I interviewed began self-pleasuring at this time, either because they were overly stimulated by encounters with the other sex or because they were so curious about the new functioning of their own bodies. And teenagers have a great capacity for self-love—teenage boys can have about eight orgasms a day, if they choose, and girls, possibly more, if they feel comfortable about their sexuality.)

Sexual values fluctuate wildly for adolescents—and this is as true today as it was thirty or forty years ago. Then we feared pregnancy, gonorrhea, and loss of respect. Today, teens fear death from HIV, if not a crippling STD that can knock out a sex life and reproductive potential forever. Some kids restrict their sexual activity to everything *but* intercourse. Ask a girl today if she is sexually active, and she may hotly argue, "Of course not! I just lie there." Lack of movement becomes a rationale for being "a good girl."

Ask a boy what he does sexually and he will admit to "messing around," but will generally go blank if asked to define an ongoing, fulfilling sexual life. Monogamy is greatly valued by some teens, scorned by others. Sexual standards for young adults are all over the map right now, as society tries to balance out the careless-sex-is-just-natural-so-why-not-do-it contingent and the restrictive total abstinence dicta of the religious right.

Homosexual experimentation is common at this age as teenagers work out their confusions about gender identity. It's sometimes easier to kiss and hug a person of your own sex because it's more like touching yourself—a known commodity. Of course, homosexual experiences can be chalked up to rebellion, but for many, it's the real thing. Sometimes, because teens fear their peers' censure, they may deny their true homosexual feelings and go for the norm. This can lead to depression, sexual dysfunction, and a lifetime of lying. It's very often only in midlife, when homosexual fantasies and desires can no longer be ignored, that people come into their true sexuality.

Those who are heterosexual, however, are now able to populate as they copulate. Males and females are technically able to conceive from the first years of pubertal development. Males can have an erection, ejaculate and have another erection within moments, sometimes stimulated only by a whiff of perfume or the sight of an appealing half-clothed body on the beach. Females can lubricate when aroused by touch or even verbal suggestion. And many can become pregnant at the drop of a condom.

Young Adulthood

Adult sexuality carries responsibility along with it. Not that every grownup is "grown up" about the way that he or she relates sexually, but most connect good sex with an expectation of solidity in a relationship. As much advertised as the "Peter Pan syndrome" (the urge to fly away from commitment) has been, the current climate advocates picking one mate at a time. This is, in part, due to the fact that promiscuous sex doesn't work any more. Even if you don't consider it morally reprehensible, you can die from it.

These expectations can lead to a lot of anxiety and sexual dysfunction. A man who sees every woman as a husband hunter may not be able to attain or maintain an erection or control his ejaculation. Paul, who had been brought up in a strict Mormon setting, had his first sex with prostitutes. He would come within fifteen minutes and spend the rest of the hour just talking. "There was nothing else at stake—I wasn't expected to act a certain way as I did around Mormon women who were supposedly 'good matches.' When I had sex with a pro, I was relaxed and felt good about myself. I could get hard again at the end of my time with them and have another orgasm and ejaculation. But it was a lot more difficult when I finally left home and met someone I liked. I was tongue-tied, and I fell all over myself trying to make her come. I couldn't begin to ask her for what I wanted."

A woman who is anxious about her sexuality will often have difficulty lubricating. If she can't be verbal with her partner, it can be difficult or even excruciating to attempt penetration. If she's constantly trying to please her partner, she may not let go enough to have an orgasm, or may fake orgasm just to get it over with. So many young women I interviewed said something like, "I had to be in love to do this," implying that they ignored their true sexual desires for the illusive warmth and comfort they could get by being with a man. Although it would seem that lesbian women would be better able to share a mutual sexuality, some reported that in early adulthood, when they tended to be partnered with an older woman who was dominant and more demanding, they couldn't stand up for themselves. They ignored their own needs, tried to please their partner, and faked orgasm just as their heterosexual counterparts did. It was only in later life that both homosexual and heterosexual women started to ask for what they wanted. Maybe this was because prior to that time, they had no idea what they wanted.

For many adults, this is a time of life when sexuality is bound up with the ideas of marriage and family. This may be equally true of gays as of straights—there are an increasing number of partnerships and adoptions in the homosexual community at this time of life.

A lot of myths pervade the arenas of marriage and sex. Some say the legitimization of a union automatically kills desire; it was juicier and hotter before, when you didn't have to spend all day every day together, when you didn't have to adjust to another's whims, desires and habits. Others find that it's hard to keep up with society's version of the "honeymoon couple," many of whom are temporarily out of commission due to acute cases of vaginitis, brought on by lack of lubrication during marathon sex sessions!

Pregnancy and Childbirth

It's a shame that men and women are primed for parenting when they are least ready to accept the emotional and financial responsibilities of raising kids—but that's nature for you. A woman is most physically fit for childbearing in her early twenties, when hormonal levels have reached their peak and every body part, from the uterus to the blood vessels, are elastic and vibrant. The younger the mother, the more capable she is physiologically to carry the burden of pregnancy and lactation. Of course, a twenty-year-old's lack of experience or her reticence about sex, or an overanxious mother-in-law may add the psychological burden of stress to conception. I always hope that succeeding generations will get smarter and wait until their thirties. But it's a slim hope.

Young men are ready to father children at any time, and often, because they are immature, they do it just to say they've done it. As testosterone levels rise, sperm production does too, and these healthy young specimens have no trouble swimming upstream to find a suitable egg to fertilize. A young man's amazing erectile function means that he may have an ejaculation and then be ready for another ten minutes to half an hour later. The possibilities for fathering children are daunting.

For many married couples, pregnancy is absolutely the best reason, the *ne plus ultra* of sex. And in fact, the closeness two people can share as they come together to create life can add a new dimension to the physical act. This is usually the first time that people report feeling a spiritual bond with their mate. One woman, now in midlife, told me she knew every time she and her husband had conceived. It was as though the energy between them locked onto one of her eggs and his sperm.

Pregnancy and sex seem to have a love–hate relationship, however. In the first trimester, when the body's hormonal status is going through rapid changes, the woman may feel too sick and tired for sex. (If there's spotting or any difficulty holding the pregnancy, the obstetrician may actually prohibit sex.) Even if women are turned off to sex in their first three months, they have an increased need for cuddling and touching, as do their partners. Massage is one of the greatest boons to pregnancy in any trimester, so a good basis for learning to touch differently is to lay on hands in a nonsexual but very sensual manner.

Some couples enter a twilight zone of no sex during this time, which can extend through the pregnancy. Because of the all-pervasive message in society that only thin is sexy, it's often difficult for a very pregnant woman to feel attractive, and her concentration on becoming a mother may block out her erotic feelings toward her husband.

But when a man finds his wife's large belly a damper on his libido, this can be more serious. He may lose his desire for sex because he can't handle the difference in what he sees and feels from the woman he married, or he may have trouble handling the connection between motherhood and sexuality. Many men are panicked about disturbing the baby within or turned off by the idea of their erotic endeavors being somehow watched or felt by the baby.

Although most ob/gyns will be happy to allay a couples' fears on this subject, superstition dies hard. There are still some prudish members of the old medical establishment who cannot tolerate the commingling of hot sex and imminent parenthood. How can the sweet mother act and feel erotic? And this type of thinking is easily passed on to parents. If one or both partners are anxious or repelled by the notion of mixing sex and the miracle of birth, professional counseling may be in order. Sex is not just a part of life in general, it is the springboard for new life. It is therefore a fitting and just pairing of excitement and arousal in a relationship and expectation of a new role as a parent for a pregnant couple to have frequent and joyous sex together.

The second trimester, when the fetus is well established in utero and the anxieties and discomforts of the first few months are over, is traditionally a wonderful time for couples. It's typical for a woman's sex drive to increase—so much so that many supplement frequent intercourse with masturbation. Many women report that they had never felt so sexual, so free. The increased blood flow to the genitalia increases sensitivity and arousal. The greater interest in sex right now is also due to beta-endorphin activity in the brain that gives an incredible feeling of well-being. The reasons are physiological and psychological—the body has balanced itself hormonally, there is no menstrual mess or discomfort, no need for contraception or planning, and, generally, a feeling of pervasive love for the person you're sharing your life with.

During the third trimester, you may reach a point where it's too cumbersome to be sexual. You can stay active longer into this trimester if you're willing to experiment with different positions and use lots of pillows. Women may have to change their postures often to avoid cramps in the legs or pelvic area, and the baby's own activity level may dictate what goes on between the partners. This is often hard on the male partner, and there are certainly enough cases of panicky fathers-to-be having extramarital affairs during this time. Problems in a marriage may be heightened by all the various changes that will occur soon after the impending birth, and should be discussed as a couple, and possibly with your doctor or a marriage and family counselor.

Are you supposed to stop being sexual just because you're about to be parents? Of course not unless yours is a high-risk pregnancy where placenta praevia or preterm rupture of the membranes would be dangerous to you or your fetus. In this case, your doctor may tell you to abstain during the last weeks. There may be health reasons that would prevent any activity (masturbation, manual or oral stimulation, or penetration) that might set off an orgasm and uterine contractions that would begin the birth process prematurely.

But in general, this is very old-fashioned thinking, brought on by the Mommy–sexpot clash of images. Enlightened physicians today feel that if sex relaxes you and reduces your stress, you should probably keep doing it as long as you and your partner are willing.

---

*S*EX *D*URING *P*REGNANCY *R*EMINDERS

- Blowing into the vagina used to be considered a risk because an air bubble carried in the bloodstream might cause embolism and stroke. Actually, there have been only eight documented cases of this unusual occurrence. Perhaps, then, better to suck than to blow at this time of life.

- It's a good idea for the woman to urinate after sex to clear the bladder and kidneys and avoid urinary tract infections.

- At any time, but especially during pregnancy, you must wash off the penis after anal sex before having vaginal intercourse. The bacteria from one area can cause an infection in the other.

Postpartum

For the first few weeks of your new child's life, sex is usually the last thing on your mind. You are too exhausted, drained, and anxious to get awfully erotic. If you are the mother, you may be sore from an episiotomy or a tear during the birth process. Your hormonal rebound will make you very dry and may reduce your libido as well. If you are the father, you are undoubtedly overwhelmed with assuming the responsibility of caring for this small dependent creature and concerned about your new relationship to the child and to your partner.

With all the sleepless nights, constant feeding, bathing, changing, and worrying, who has the time or the inclination to make love? As soon as you take off your clothes and climb into bed, you fall asleep!

But generally after your third week, if there is no more postpartum bleeding, you're both fit enough for anything—all you have to do is stay awake. (Some couples prefer to wait until the sixth-week gynecological checkup for an okay from their physician.) You and your partner should start slowly, of course, with massage, gentle touching, and just as much stimulation of the genital area—with lubrication as necessary—as you're up to.

If you are nursing, you may have an experience of arousal and, for some, actual orgasm, as your baby sucks at your nipple. This is not wrong, perverted, or bizarre. The body puts out a hormone called *oxytocin* (known as the "let-down hormone") during intercourse, during the birth process, and during lactation. Orgasm triggers the release when you're sexually active; the suckling of an infant—sometimes just the crying of your infant—causes it to flow and let the milk down. At the same time, you may experience uterine contractions. So it's very much like sex. Your partner can do the same for you, if you both wish, by stimulating your nipples. Many men are very turned on by the idea of sampling mother's milk. If you think it's too weird, you can always express a little into a spoon and give a taste that way.

Remember: You feel sexier after the birth of your child. Pregnancy brings an increase in the volume of blood flow through the pelvis, and this in turn increases your capacity for sexual tension, orgasmic intensity, and frequency.

Male Sexual Changes During the Thirties and Forties

While women are on the baby track, men in their thirties and early forties are more concerned with sexual prowess. If they're not married, they are undoubtedly juggling the issues of "getting enough" and staying disease-free at the same time. They may be anxious with a new partner (or a string of new partners) and find that they ejaculate too quickly to make a sexual encounter a long, delicious affair. They are also arriving at a point where they aren't quite as prolific—though a twenty-year-old may have over one hundred orgasms a year, by age forty, the number has dwindled to a mere eighty. No longer do men at this stage wake with an erection each morning, and in most cases, their erections have drooped from above to below the horizontal.

After the age of thirty-five, when the body has reached its natural peak, all systems start slowing down. Testosterone levels decrease slightly, as do the number of spermatozoa released in each ejaculation as well as the various secretions from the prostate and seminal vesicles. Although these physiological changes have absolutely nothing to do with a man's sexual awareness or enjoy-ment, they give many men the willies. Does it mean you can't per-form if you perform differently? Certainly not.

But suppose you are in a married relationship and are contem-plating a family. Many men are besieged with terrible fear, once con-traception has been abandoned, that they won't be able to deliver the goods. Infertility is more widespread among couples today, par-ticularly since a great number of them wait until their careers are established before starting a family. When the kids don't come along with the greatest of ease, men are subjected to one test after anoth-er, and are often swept up in the complex and highly structured game of "let's make a baby" that takes all the joy out of sex.

The often futile tests, temperature taking, and precise times of the month can make men despair, and can often lead to erectile dys-function. When you are expected to perform, very often you don't feel like it. A great deal of stress can depress your endorphin levels, which in turn can decrease testosterone levels. And there you have a particularly vicious cycle. Heavy stress in a man of this age is a real risk factor for heart attack and other serious physical problems.

Men in their thirties and forties can be, of course, at the peak of their sexual capacity, particularly in the context of a warm and giving monogamous relationship. Continued interest in a partner very often results from a sense of bonding—from two, becoming one.

Menopause and Women's Midlife Changes

Women's first indication of a shift in their sexuality usually comes around the perimenopause, which can occur anywhere from age thirty-eight to fifty-three. Women still need to use contraception until at least eighteen months after their final period if they aren't interested in continuing their family, but after that, they can breathe a sigh of relief and separate sexual pleasure from reproductive anx-iety. Even during the perimenopause, most women have a depleted supply of eggs, and those that do remain in the ovaries are usually unfit to become fertilized.

Somewhere in the mid- to late forties, estrogen levels start to drop dramatically, and this means a decline in the juiciness of the tissues. After age forty-eight or so, the number of layers of epithelial tissue in a woman's vagina shrinks, and this thinner skin is more susceptible to irritation or infection. Less estrogen means less lubrication, even when aroused.

Can this detract from feeling sexy? You bet. The biggest complaint from women who have enjoyed their sex life prior to menopause is that awful dry feeling, even when they're aroused (and with aging, there is an overall decrease in the excitement phase leading to orgasm anyway). Lubrication before and during sex is an absolute necessity for most women at this time of life, with or without a partner.

We are less elastic all over as we age, and the vaginal opening is one area that loses a great deal of springiness, again, due to the reduced amount of estrogen. But if we're willing to work at it and add a little variety to our sexual activities, we can achieve orgasms that are just as rich and long-lasting—sometimes moreso—than those we enjoyed in younger days. Breasts that are stimulated and suckled will retain their allure and excitement, even if they're more pendulous than they used to be. They aren't as perky simply because the percentage of fat tissue to muscle tissue declines over time. But so what?

Hot flashes, the physical evidence of our hormonal imbalance, have no effect on sexuality. Reports from most women, however, say they are never oblivious to flashes and they tend to make them less desirous of sex, because, when you're sweating buckets anyway, do you really want to participate in an activity that is going to produce even more perspiration? Estrogen replacement (discussed shortly) can be a libido enhancer partly because it tends to reduce flashing. It also nearly doubles vaginal blood flow after just one month of therapy, and this, too, leads to improved sexual function.

What else happens to a woman when she gets older? That lovely flush around the breasts and labia that occurred when you were aroused doesn't happen as easily. The labia don't change color—they used to go from pink to burgundy—and the uterus doesn't lift up as it used to. The size of the clitoris decreases, and the clitoral hood isn't as full, nor is the mons pubis as nicely padded with fat tissue.

Orgasms may trigger fewer uterine contractions as we age, but the feeling is usually just as intense as it used to be. Women can have multiple orgasms as they get older and more experienced and discover how they can be in charge mentally as well as physically (see Questions and Answers About Orgasm, Chapter Eleven). In the resolution stage, the clitoris quickly retracts from its tumescent state (just as the male penis does!).

Do these changes really make a difference? In a variety of studies on sexual response in older women, it was reported that desire for sex decreased by over half, but enjoyment of the sexual act decreased only by a quarter. And the ease of achieving orgasm, too, went down by only 25 percent. The frequency of fantasizing didn't change much over the years. The parameters of change in this study indicated that it wasn't just all the stuff going on in the body that might have been unsettling or confusing that made the women want less sex. Very often, it was the marital status of the respondent!

Women didn't want sex as much when their male partners gave them less time to use lubrication or didn't feel the need for increased touching, kissing, cuddling—all the things that used to be called "foreplay," but which we now acknowledge as anytime play. Studies show that there is a marked difference in hormonal output in women when they initiate sex from when they just passively receive a partner's attention. This is one more good reason to keep sexually active at this time of life.

Single women tended to feel better about their bodies as they got older and, of course, the stimulation of having a partner who hasn't seen you every day, good times and bad for the last twenty or thirty years, might have had something to do with the freshness of their sex life. Lesbians, by the way, had fewer declines in all four areas, possibly because they had partners who understood what they were going through.

How to Stay Sexually Fit at Midlife

Communicate Your New Needs to Your Partner

There is a vicious cycle going on in midlife bedrooms. Many women are embarrassed to stop and ask a partner to use saliva or a water-based lubricant before they dive right in, and this means increased anxiety, which means lowered natural lubrication, which means difficult sex. The act of penetration can actually become agonizing or impossible due to psychological and physical factors.

Is it becoming clear why communication between partners is so essential? If you can't ask for a lube job, you can't ask for love.

Lubricate Thoroughly and Frequently

KY Jelly is the standard water-based lubricant, but there are now many new brands on the market, such as Astroglide, Probe, GyneMoistrin, and Replens. They are available in drugstores and supermarkets. Condoms that are pretreated with nonoxynol-9 will also add some slippery enhancement.

Though it might have taken a few seconds to feel wet during the reproductive years, it may take an older woman four to five minutes to become aroused, and she may still feel terribly dry. Believe me when I say that it is more enjoyable for both partners when you both are comfortable, and whether the topic is using a condom or moistening your fingers with saliva, it's essential to stop and *say* the words.

Lubrication problems typically are more virulent in women who have been less sexually active over the years. Let the following thought ring in your consciousness: *You must use it or lose it.* This is particularly true if you don't have a partner at menopause due to divorce or death or you desire a period of celibacy. If you ever anticipate having a sexual encounter involving intercourse again, you must take care of yourself now by masturbating, preferably with a dildo or vibrator. If you don't, and months pass without any stimulation in that area, it will be increasingly difficult to introduce even a finger, let alone a penis, should you wish to in the future.

Do Kegel Exercises

To keep the perineal area fit, there is nothing like *Kegel exercises* (named for the doctor who invented them). It's incredibly easy to master these vital internal squeezes.

Think about urinating and then muscularly stopping the flow of urine and you've got it. What you are squeezing are the *pubococcygeal muscles (PC muscles)*, as well as the *anal sphincter muscles*. When you become really expert, you will be able to divide the two and exercise one set at a time. Most doctors recommend three sets of ten Kegels, performed three times a day. You should practice them both slowly and quickly.

If you have trouble with the technique, introduce a finger into your vagina and squeeze around it, holding it tight. You'll be able to feel if you're letting up the pressure, and when your muscle tone is getting stronger.

Kegels can be performed while you're chopping vegetables or waiting on line at the bank. They can save you from late-life incontinence as well as increasing the pleasure you give yourself and your partner as you wrap yourself around whatever's inside you.

Men's Midlife Changes

Men don't experience the dramatic drop in gonadal hormones that women do, but that doesn't mean they aren't affected by the changes that do occur. What concerns they have about performance, about how big their erections are today as compared to yesterday, how long they can go in bed! There is nothing (I've been told over and over) like not being as hard as you used to be. On the other hand, there's nothing to do about it but to agree, with your partner, to try new things and have fun in your new shape and size.

Yes, it does take longer for a man in midlife to get a firm erection when aroused, and it may be harder to maintain. But ask any heterosexual woman what she likes from her partner in bed, and she'll never mention the erection first. What she wants, and now can have because her partner requires it, is more time for sexual activities other than intercourse.

There are some other physiological changes worth mentioning: The angle of the erection is lower, as is the whole scrotum. Many men fear that their penis is shrinking over time—in fact, it's an optical illusion because their scrotal sac hangs lower. (After holding the testes up for fifty years or so, it naturally drops.) The orgasm itself is over more quickly, the force and volume of the ejaculate are less, and the penis becomes flaccid sooner after climax. The refractory period (that is, the time between one ejaculation and the next firm erection that might lead to another ejaculation) may run from several hours to an entire day.

This saddens younger men greatly and often makes them dread the aging process. Yet there's such a range of sexuality to consider from licking, sucking, kissing, rubbing, touching, thinking and talking, laughing, and talking some more—so who needs another erection right away? The idea of having to be hard all the time goes back to that old conservative notion that sex is all about sticking one body part inside another. This is outdated rubbish. A healthy, desirous older man can have sex constantly, round the clock. He simply can't always have it with a stiff penis.

Is there a male "viropause" or "andropause"? This is a tricky question, and I personally think the answer is no if you're comparing it to the female menopause. There are doctors out there advocating testosterone replacement for men, but they are in the distinct minority. Yes, about a third of all men experience a decline in their testosterone levels after fifty, but it is *not* lowered testosterone that is predictive of erectile dysfunction. Actually, another androgen, DHEAS (dihydroepiandrosterone sulfate), is the culprit here, and it may also be implicated in the development of cardiovascular disease.

Most of the drop in male testosterone levels takes place over the long haul, from the ages of about sixty to one hundred. But men are fertile throughout their lifespan barring any illness or surgery that removes or damages their androgen output—Picasso and Casals fathered children when they were in their eighties. Men are also fortunate in that their biochemical and physical changes (loss of elasticity of tissue, decline in muscle mass) are usually so slow and gradual as to be imperceptible to the unpracticed eye.

Men do experience big emotional changes as they age, but many of them deny it. Their sense of power, be it in their career, their family, their personal life, is so bound up with ego and personality that it can be devastating to feel little bits of it slowly slipping away. A man in midlife who takes a younger partner may start to suffer from fear of failure in bed—but is the real concern about possibly not pleasing her, or is it terror of the image of aging we are stuck with—the awful specter of senescence and decrepitude? To conquer these fears, men must start getting in touch with the deeper core of their true effectiveness, the part of their being that doesn't depend on being big, fast, tough, or in charge. They can do this only if they are willing to keep an open mind about their worth and their real capacities.

Resetting Your Sexual Clock with Hormone Replacement Therapy and Androgen Therapy

Here are a few words about hormone replacement therapy. The prevailing thought in the medical arena these days is that you should be considering the notion of replacing estrogen and progesterone, the hormones that are depleted with aging (unless you've had an estrogen-dependent cancer).

Because estrogen affects over three hundred tissues in the body, many signs and symptoms—some of which are menopausal and some of which are due to the natural aging process—can be forestalled by taking supplemental hormones. Wide-scale short-term studies (the longest of these only go ten years out) show that estrogen replacement protects the heart, the bones, the genitourinary structures, and the skin, and it also interacts with other hormones that allow us to deal with emotional and physical stress. Hot flashes and vaginal dryness are usually ameliorated, if not alleviated, by hormone replacement therapy (HRT).

But there's a flip side, too. To really protect yourself from heart attack and osteoporosis ("porous bones"), you should ideally stay on this medication as long as you have a heart and bones, that is, until death do you part. But putting a substance into the body for so many years at a time of life when absorption of medication is not always as easy to monitor as it is in a younger person, presents some considerable problems.

HRT-takers put themselves at a higher risk for endometrial and, possibly, breast cancers, and there are other risks, including liver and gallbladder disease, high blood pressure, and radical mood swings. Because every body is different, and some are exquisitely sensitive to amounts and types of estrogen and progesterone, dosages should be very precisely titrated, but most physicians don't take the time or don't have the pharmacological expertise to do this. Often, women aren't told exactly why and how to take HRT and may slack off after less than a year.

The question of whether or not to take HRT will be debated hotly for years to come. Does it make a difference in your sexuality? Estrogen can make you more comfortable physically by improving vaginal acidity levels and increasing fluid and blood flow to the genitals. But progestins can wreak havoc with your libido and give you PMS symptoms to boot. Small doses of androgens (the male sex hormone) may bring back sex drive or increase it, but they can't fix a broken marriage. Other hormones, considerably less studied than estrogen and progesterone, also decrease as we age, and no one is sure how these affect sexuality. A loving, caring partner or a new exciting one may have far more impact on desire and lubrication than HRT.

Older Sex Opens up New Dimensions

Everybody alive—regardless of their age—is afraid of getting old. I am, too. I'm worried about how I'll feel, how I'll look, and what I'll lose as I age.

I confess this trepidation about getting older because I am such a staunch proponent of sexuality for older individuals. When I say older, I'm not talking midlife, I'm speaking of those from 80 on up, a developmental stage I call *highlife*. Because I see myself remaining a hot, active, juicy woman even as I wrinkle and grow slightly shorter and have decreasing stores of estrogen to give me a sense of well-being and a lowered testosterone level that may make it more difficult for my libido to sing.

A lot of people have trouble with the image of a sexually active older person. The "dirty old man" or "dirty old lady" is made into a joke instead of congratulated for having such a wonderful time for so many years. Jack, a concert pianist in his thirties, told me, "I can see myself being sexy at eighty. My problem is I can't begin to imagine myself making love to an eighty-year-old." In the past, the picture of an individual in advanced old age was completely asexual. It's time to change that image.

In highlife, deeper aspects of our sexuality come into play. Maybe the peaks in a relationship start to coincide with the maturity or the integration of a coupled relationship. In older individuals, whose bond has survived the ravages of time, there is less need to exert power, to maintain an attitude, to use sex when other avenues of communication fail.

Alex, on his third marriage at seventy, said, "My second wife and I were incredibly sexual together; my third wife doesn't like sex much, and I've adjusted. Even though she doesn't like to be penetrated, she does enjoy it when I stimulate her manually and when she does the same for me. I don't feel I'm missing anything. I know what's out there, after all. But she and I enjoy so many other things together, I think I've learned to use the feelings I got from sex in other ways."

Heidi, a former city planner of seventy-four, said she now thinks of herself as a "sexual guru," making the awareness of herself as a sexual being helpful to others that she mentors. And Abram, a medical writer of sixty-two with hypertension, said that he tended to get more attention from younger women than he ever did. "I want to follow up, you know, because I have just as much curiosity as before, but hey, the idea of explaining all that about not having erections is too much of a pain in the butt. So I deflect the interest another way, and I flirt and get close and touch, and tend to enjoy the women anyway."

Touch, getting close. Here's the ticket. The longer we maintain that skin and eye contact with others, the longer we are keyed into this healing energy that steams up the windows. Teenagers jump into bed, or into the backseat of cars, because it's fun, it's expected, to fit in, to avoid breaking up, for money, because they can't control themselves, because—just sometimes—it feels good. Rarely are they physically and emotionally ready for the heady experience of clicking with another individual when desire meets *understanding*.

As we proceed in life, we may find ourselves in sexual relationships because we wish to yield or wield power, because we crave a little less loneliness, because we want to make an impression, because we want to make a family—all kinds of reasons spark our desire.

But the aging process itself prepares us for another kind of sexuality, that which has a basis in the whole life of the person. When the body is no longer the clever trickster it used to be, and the mind is filled with more memories than expectations, we are ready to move toward another human being from a position of greater self-awareness.

Patience comes with age, and this is a benefit because everything takes longer, for both men and women. You have to be gentle with the sexual organs—they are thinner now, with less fat padding, and should be handled carefully. Some older women may leak a little urine when the penis presses on the uterus which in turn presses on the bladder. But there are remedies for stress incontinence—one of the best is doing the Kegel exercises recommended earlier in this chapter. Women of this age may not be as interested in intercourse, but most still crave intimacy. This can mean many things to many different people.

Let us take the case of Lois, an eighty-three-year-old great grandmother. She's in good physical condition, but has difficulty walking, so she can't always get to the kitchen to prepare food for herself. Her family wants her in a safe place, so they convince her to move into a nursing home. Now here's a woman, widowed for fifteen years, who has been treated with kindness and indulgence by her relatives for quite a while. She's not really been looked at as "Lois" for a long time, but as "grandma." But in the nursing home, she is suddenly on her own socially, and it is a revelation to her.

Two men, both about a decade younger than she, begin to pay her court, and Larry, the younger man, is really determined. He is a good talker, a lover of books and movies, someone who learned she collected chess sets and bought her a small set she could put in her pocketbook. He is a pal, a man who likes himself and feels at ease extending himself to others.

Over the weeks, as she and Larry get more intimate, they are seen holding hands in public, their bodies close, Larry matching his gait to her slower one when they walk. One evening, she invites him into her room, and they lie down on her bed, hugging and fondling one another for an hour, although they don't take their clothes off. Lois reports feeling enormously comfortable with this man, unselfconscious about her physical limitations, relaxed and giving of her entire self, not just her body parts. She has no particular desire for sexual intercourse, but as their relationship proceeds, and it's clear that Larry wants it, she agrees. She does not reach orgasm when Larry is inside her, but she does, occasionally, have a brief peak of excitement that she describes as "the lights going on," through manual stimulation.

Bernard D. Starr and Marcella B. Weiner conducted an extensive survey on attitudes of older people toward sexuality and they found that most older men and women felt sex was important for both physical and emotional health, that it could improve with age, that variety was important, that nudity was enjoyable, that living together outside traditional marriage was okay. Forty percent said that orgasm was an essential part of the sexual experience, and most seemed to be having them regularly, because they claimed satisfaction with their sex lives.

One of the biggest problems of sexuality and aging is the lack of partners. Women typically live six and a half years longer than men, so if they were hooked up heterosexually with one individual for most of a lifetime, it can be difficult, if not impossible, to find themselves coupled in later life. (Since women often marry men older than themselves, they may be in midlife when this problem begins.) So many more women over sixty-five means competition for male partners, or as is increasingly the case, a decision to select another female partner.

Gay and Lesbian Couples in Later Life

In our homophobic society, it is still incredibly difficult to come out as a homosexual and live comfortably with or without a partner within the context of a heterosexual world. But as gays and lesbians get older, there are sometimes more options and more freedom.

During midlife, where many married partners are coming apart at the seams, gay and lesbian couples are finding community. There are formal and informal groups that may live close to one another and meet at the same restaurants, bars, bookstores, and so forth. The typical physical and emotional changes of aging, though sometimes very difficult for gay men who have prided themselves on their looks and build, are not looked on with such dismay in the lesbian community. Women accept women's bodies when they are not preening to achieve some artificial standard of beauty. Whereas two-income lesbian couples may earn less collectively than two-income heterosexual or gay couples, they are usually in better shape in terms of their cooperative financial picture. It is not common for one partner to expect the other—or their children—to look after them in their old age. They are generally more equal partners in life and in bank accounts.

They are also usually more comfortable with their aging sexuality. As Hannah put it, "We're whole people together, whether we're standing kissing in the kitchen or taking a walk by the pond. My partner's sexual energy and mine have come together after all these years—what we're doing is *living* as a couple, not eating, sleeping, making love, doing the taxes as a couple. Sex doesn't exist in a vacuum; our need to express our sexuality to one another is just part of a need to reassure one another that we're here and in love."

How to Get Your Sexual Rhythms in Sync with Your Partner's

No matter your age or developmental stage, there are times when you feel like it, and your partner doesn't. And vice versa. And there are times when you are both ambivalent.

A good way to get more in sync is to try some other exercises that make your actions and feelings coincide:

- Breathe or meditate together (see Chapter Ten).
- Go ballroom dancing together.
- Swim together.
- Sing songs or make music together in harmony.
- Go to sleep and wake up together.

When you want to work up to sexual timing compatibility, you have to take a number of elements into consideration. For example,

1. *Are you a lark and is your partner an owl?* You must compromise if you are a lark living with an owl. Larks rise with the sun or before and find most of their energy high early in the day, and owls don't wake up until noon and are most energetic at night. When one of you loves sex in the early light of dawn and the other is dead to the world, try meeting in the afternoon.

2. *Do you have a schedule for your sex life?* This is *not* to say that you must pencil in times of the week on your filofax and have your secretary confirm the appointment. According to Winnifred Cutler, Ph.D., author of *Love Cycles,* sexual activity on a weekly basis (it can be more frequent if you wish!) promotes a regular cycle for women and higher sperm viability for men. Partnered activity enhances these capacities more than masturbation.

3. *Do you use the power of your sex attractants? Pheromones* are the chemical substances produced in the glands like hormones. A

hormone acts as a chemical messenger within the body; a pheromone acts as a messenger between two bodies. You can't "smell" a particular scent that makes your partner desirable to you, but the pheromones present in sweat and body secretions from the pores (armpits and upper lips are highly attracting areas) actually influence what goes on between you. You can consciously allow your natural essences to work by getting rid of heavy perfumes and aftershaves and scented deodorants. Snuggling up in the crook of your partner's underarm or rubbing under her nose may do wonders for your sex life!

Accept Changes in Your Sexuality

Think of yourself sitting in a sunlit glen on a fall afternoon with the breeze blowing the branches around.

Just like sex, in you and in the air at the same time.

You are reading a book which is alternately kissed by sunlight or shaded by clouds.

Just like sex, sometimes clear, sometimes obscure to you.

You squint, then your eyes level out as the glare retreats. You get a whiff of the powerful smell of decaying leaves, then an odor of green grass prevails. Then, as the wind stills, no smell.

Just like sex, it's there and it's not there, simultaneously. It contains your creative, social, and healing energies as well as your instinctive drive toward physical release.

Your sexuality is very much akin to this experience—you simply have to be aware of its changes because it doesn't hit like a blast of wind or a blinding ray of sun. But every moment of your life, as your body goes through its various hormonal and neuronal changes, you are changing into a slightly different sexual being. Tapping into those changes will expand your repertoire, and alter the way you think about yourself. You will find a sexual core that runs throughout your day, your month, your life—one that you can always tap into for nourishment.

How to Get More Good Sex into Your Busy Life

*I*f you could make all your fantasies come true, would you have sex all the time? Never? Only when you were feeling physically well? Are there times when it's not so desirable to have sex? How do you know? Thomas, a widower in his eighties who was sexually active until his wife's death last year, told me how wonderful he used to feel on Sunday mornings after he and his wife had their Saturday night "date." The glow always lasted until the next day. For him, Saturday night was the "right" time.

They had a specific schedule, a time, a place, and a few tried and true positions. Spontaneity was the one thing they lacked.

And yet, because sex is such a surprise every time we venture into it, it is worthwhile noting that there are many appropriate times to have sex—and some, when we feel like having sex, that are not so appropriate. By being sensitive to your moods and your partner's, you will increase your sexuality time management immeasurably.

Can You Heal a Bad Argument with Good Sex?

People fight and make up. If they didn't, they wouldn't be able to sustain a relationship for very long. Some couples thrive on battle—it charges them up, gives them that extra edge that is very often sexual.

When we have an argument, we rise to an emotional peak. We're in a state of high tension and high arousal. Everything seems crucial and urgent, and the qualities we value in a partner are suddenly thrown into a very harsh light. But we would never be *this* angry at a person we didn't care about—it's hard to get worked up when there isn't much at stake. Nancy, a passionate thirty-seven-year-old beautician who admits her high threshold for intense personal involvement, said succinctly, "I don't know what it is about me and Alan, but when we're not fucking, we're fighting."

164

Yet it's very common to do both. How often have you had a major blowup that has ended either in a surly truce or an impulsive need to get away from your partner before you hit her or him? (People who cross the line are in serious need of therapy or counseling. The number of battered wives in this country is staggering and increases daily, and the syndrome unfortunately manifests itself in a cooperation between batterer and batteree—the couple always forgive and forget—until next time, which sadly may be the last time.)

One way of redirecting anger before it becomes violent is to take that physical impetus into sex. So many people told me that they often made up in the bedroom, having some of the wildest, most rewarding sex they'd ever experienced.

But I don't think the bedroom is the best place for this kind of negotiation. Unless you've talked honestly about your real feelings of explosive anger beforehand, you haven't tackled the problem directly. When you move your rage into the physical realm of sex, you are taking the sexual experience and turning it into a power struggle. In fact, this is exactly what rape is—the domination of one person by another to work out overwhelming feelings of impotence and helplessness on the part of the attacker. It is not, therefore, a good idea to use the impetus for conflict as a jump-off point for intimacy. It confuses the very delicate issues a couple faces daily.

Who's on top? Who leads and who follows? is one of the primary foci of couples' sharing. Here's a list of questions to ask *before* you go into the bedroom:

1. Who gets his or her way most of the time?
2. How are arguments begun and ended?
3. When you feel "stirred up," do you want to take it out on someone physically?
4. Is it difficult for you to become aroused and therefore desirous of a sexual encounter? Does anger help to get your energy—and tension level—up?
5. What other ways could you resolve your differences that would generate energy but give you time to talk? (Making dinner or going for a bike ride together, raking leaves or throwing snowballs at each other.)
6. What transition or ritual could you devise to bridge the time between being angry and being loving?

The more aware you are of your natural reactions to bad feelings, the easier it will be to translate your tension into positive activities. You can benefit yourself and your partner by accepting all the hot, excited feelings you have and directing them elsewhere for a while. Sex to fix a fight is not a good idea; but allowing your sexuality into the making-up process is an excellent notion.

How to Balance Your Love Life and the Real World

We all have a fantasy of being able to run off to Tahiti with the one we want to be most intimate with. We'd lie naked on our own beach, enjoying the weather, the water, and each other. We'd offer tidbits of breadfruit and mango, interspersed with incredible sex. We'd breathe easy all the time when we weren't panting with lust.

But there is no Tahiti in real life. Interruptions are a part of everyone's daily routine. We must be able to keep our own focus and persevere, even if the phone is ringing off the hook, the work is piling up and everything conspires to interfere with your sex life. A set of visiting in-laws or friends, an *au pair* or tenant who shares your home, a long-running appearance of workmen around the house, or the perennial patter of feet (children's or neighbors') will kill that urge before it takes wing.

How do you handle it? How do you make space for all the intrusions of the real world in your love life?

- Be prepared to be unprepared. Take the moments you get and revel in them. It can be exciting to make love hurriedly, so desperate for one another that you don't even make time to take most of your clothes off.

- Let children know that privacy is important. They should be taught at the earliest age possible that when the bedroom door is closed, it's off-limits (this goes for their bedroom door, too, by the way).

- Workmen are pretty diligent about lunch breaks and daily schedules. Coordinate yours to theirs.

- If your live-in guests or *au pair* don't get the message, and simply refuse to take a day off and go somewhere else, you may have to ask them directly for some free time.

- If your life is so crowded with people and events that you say you have no time for sex, there is something seriously wrong. Yes, of course you are tired at the end of a long day; yes, certainly you have clients who call at home or demand your work-time off-hours, yes, you owe your kids an afternoon of touch football or a walk around a museum, but *you still have to make time for yourself*.

Personal privacy is your birthright, and you must do everything in your power to protect it. Relationships have foundered on the cold seas of abstinence. The right time to make love is the time you protect and cherish together. This often takes devious machinations and lots of planning. But it can be fun!

Exciting Sexual Rendezvous— Six Ways to Find the Time

1. If your home is occupied, take a car ride and make love in the backseat.

2. If you are too exhausted to be sexual at bedtime, set the clock an hour earlier and wake each other with hot kisses.

3. If you notice your partner entering the shower, join him and get wet (and other things) together.

4. Take a break from weekend chores together and instead of stopping for a cup of coffee in the kitchen, stop for an erotic romp on top of the dryer.

5. Meet for lunch during the workweek at a park and throw down a blanket in a secluded area (even if you can't take off your clothes, you can have fun).

6. Set aside a cookie jar to save up for occasional jaunts to a bed-and-breakfast or even a no-tell motel on the highway.

Diet doctors have told us for years that we shouldn't be fixated on three square meals a day—it's healthier to graze like animals, taking a little here and there whenever we're really hungry, not sitting down at a table just because the clock informs us that it's mealtime. The same should be your new attitude about what the sexual experience means to you. Why at night? Why once a month, a week, a day? Sure it's wonderful to have a whole evening of flowers, music, bubble baths, and intense gazing into one another's eyes. It's also okay to shake it up a bit—find time when you are really sexually stimulated and do something about it. *Despite* the kids, the mothers-in-law, and the roofers.

Releasing Grief:
How Sex Can Help Heal You After Emotional Trauma

Grief, like anger, is a devastating emotion. It washes over us and consumes us, sometimes blocking out the rest of the world. When you are in the midst of a grieving experience, be it due to a death, a separation, a divorce, or a job loss, it can seem hard enough to become interested in yourself, let alone another individual.

And yet, it has been found that the expression of the deepest parts of our sexuality can have an enormously healing effect. When we feel another's arms around us, it is a harkening back to the beginnings of our conscious life, when we were held by loving parents. The power of touch is extraordinary—trial programs with children in a German orphanage where they were assigned one individual who would hold them and interact with them like a parent showed just how significant this experience is. The children who lacked touch were often mentally and emotionally disturbed and exhibited pathological head-banging and rocking behavior. The children who were touched often and well developed normally and, over time, were increasingly able to interact with other children and adults.

So, too with a person suffering from grief. The process of grieving is a necessary one, taking us from bargaining to denial to anger to depression to grief to mourning and finally to acceptance. The process may stop anywhere along the line, and we can get stuck in patterns of feeling and behavior that are counterproductive. We may even cross the borderline between grieving and depression if we can't get help or help ourselves. By opening up sufficiently to let in another's sexual touch, we may short-circuit the potential dangers of relinquishing everything to our sorrow.

This type of sexual experience will undoubtedly be very different in action and effect than most. A couple will most likely experience functional problems—a woman may not lubricate or be able to have an orgasm, for example, or a man may have a lot of difficulty achieving and maintaining an erection. It's important for both people to recognize that none of this difficulty is deliberate—nobody's withholding pleasure from the other on purpose. Rather, the psychological barriers to letting go and relaxing enough to "feel sexy" may be too strong. Guilt also plays a big part—how awful to feel pleasure when someone has died or when you're going through a painful break.

Yet the *connection* you make that takes you outside yourself and allows you to give and take with someone else is the linchpin to healing. Allow it, let it in, even if it's just a time to lie beside your partner and hold on for dear life.

Sex During Menstruation: Should You or Shouldn't You?

Menstruation is a mysterious and significant time of the month that can enhance each woman's sexuality. What a marvelous demonstration of the healthy, structured functioning of the human body. Of course, this terrific event has been steeped in so much taboo for so many centuries, it is understandable that people shy away from acting in a sexual way during a period. And yet, this time in a woman's cycle can open both men and women to some exciting sexual possibilities.

Most women interviewed for this book said that they usually felt hornier when they were menstruating, but even if they didn't, that sex (like exercise) relieved their cramps. (Menstrual cramps are primarily caused by an excess of prostaglandins, which will fluctuate as will many hormones and enzymes, during arousal and orgasm.) Their biggest concerns were making a mess, turning off their partner, and what kind of contraception was appropriate during a period.

Most men interviewed said they didn't mind sex during a period, but no one was wildly enthusiastic. In general, they skirted the subject of being turned off. Although no one confessed to thinking it was gross or unsettling to dip his penis into a well of blood, the idea as just phrased gave several people pause. "It's just because she's so self-conscious," one man said, getting himself off the hook at the expense of his girlfriend. "Actually, we never discussed it, but if she says she's having cramps, she's always in a terrible mood so we rarely end up doing it around then."

The only people I talked to who prohibited sex during menses were those who'd been raised in an Orthodox Jewish family. In this tradition, as in the Islamic and Hindu faiths and several others, a woman is still considered an outcast during her menses because she is thought of as "unclean." In ancient times, bleeding women in many cultures lived apart from the communal group, weren't allowed to participate in certain ceremonies, and weren't allowed to cook certain dishes, because the chef's state of body/mind during these five days was suspect.

Why were people so afraid of menstruating women? The lack of cleanliness was certainly a big issue, but other groups separated women from the group for more mystical reasons. Since a woman's cycle waxes and wanes with the moon and tides, there was a reverence for a woman's blood time, when she was ripe to receive the sacred wisdom that came from nature or the Goddess. Since women living in a group tend to cycle together because of their coordinated pheromones (see Chapter Eight), they were at the same point energetically and creatively. Typically, communally dwelling women would bleed around the dark of the moon, just before the new moon. We fear the dark because of its unknown qualities. And so women at the time were feared, for the power they could wield together.

To return to the more concrete realm of the body, what is going on physiologically during menses is a big drop in both estrogen and progesterone. Estrogen, which proliferates during the first half of a woman's cycle, has been supplanted after ovulation by a surge of progesterone, which often has an inhibiting quality on the vagina, making it dry and unreceptive to arousal. This hormone can also produce "the blues," a really low emotional state toward the end of the cycle. (In extreme cases, the anxiety and tension a woman goes through at this time are classified as PMS, or premenstrual syndrome.)

During the five to seven days where the ovarian hormonal stimuli are temporarily reduced so that the lining of the uterus can slough off, a woman may in fact feel aroused (her testosterone level, which is responsible for her libido, remains high in most women, although some do have monthly peaks that coincide with their estrogen peaks), but have trouble lubricating. And that dichotomy in desire and arousal may trigger the old cautionary statement, "Not tonight, dear."

Winnifred Cutler, Ph.D., who has written and researched a great deal in the field of endocrinology, is quite precise on the subject of hormones and horniness. In her book, *Love Cycles*, she recommends abstinence during menses for purely physiological health reasons. We know that some women suffer from retrograde menstruation—that is, an inward rather than an outward flow.

When the reproductive system is working properly, it does its monthly job of flushing out all the impurities, old blood and tissue and mucus. The experience of receiving ejaculate into the vaginal canal, however, can interrupt this outward flow. The female reproductive tract can draw sperm upward via mechanical contractions and may, as well, suck other bodily fluids backward toward the Fallopian tubes. According to Cutler, it is possible that those women who are highly susceptible to autoimmune reactions might increase their chances of developing endometriosis, a disease where the tissue that should be expelled during menses adheres to the internal organs.

But this is not a provable hypothesis, since many women do enjoy lots of sexual activity while they're bleeding and never develop any problems.

What may be a reasonable caution is to use as much protection as possible during a menstrual period, particularly for nonmonogamous couples, or couples who've known each other for only a few months. Since we know that the HIV virus is passed through blood and blood products, it's essential to have condoms and dental dams on hand and to use them for every sexual encounter. And whether you use a diaphragm for contraceptive purposes or not, you can use one during a menstrual period to contain the flow of blood.

The individual couple is the only arbiter of whether it's right or wrong to be sexual at this time. Some women love to make love when they're menstruating and just need a little lubricant to help them along. Some men don't find the blood offensive—or at least, it doesn't stop them from desiring sexual relations. Wear a diaphragm, keep a towel under you, keep tissues by the bed, stock up on condoms if you don't know each other well—and relax.

Is Sexual Dysfunction in Your Mind or Body?

It is cruel and unusual to place blame for sexual problems, so thank God it's now considered politically incorrect to do so. In the bad old days, a man who couldn't get it up all the time was "impotent" and a woman was "frigid" if she didn't want it. These is fightin' words—after all, there are those who aren't particularly interested in sex (certainly, that's their prerogative!) or have sexual problems that might stem from some trauma they suffered in the past.

Usually, it is a mix of physical, emotional, and psychological factors that combine to make sex difficult or impossible. And if one partner is having trouble, the other may respond in kind.

I talked about improving your sexual health by getting rid of alcohol, nicotine and recreational drugs in Chapter Five. But let me once again mention that abuse of any mind-altering substance as well as certain medications may cause any of the dysfunctions listed in the accompanying box. If it is within your power, or your physician's, to reduce or eliminate drug usage or change dosages or the particular medications themselves, do so. It will help your sex life immeasurably.

*F*ACTS ABOUT SEXUAL DYSFUNCTION

MALE DIFFICULTIES	POSSIBLE CAUSE
Lack of Arousal:	anger, boredom, conflict in relationship
Clinical impotence: (a man is unable to achieve and maintain an erection hard enough for penetration and ejaculation during three out of four attempts)	physical or emotional

(continued on next page)

MALE DIFFICULTIES	POSSIBLE CAUSE
Occasional difficulty achieving and/or maintaining an erection:	physical (illness or injury) or emotional (new partner).
Premature ejaculation:	inability to maintain control over stimulus that leads to "point of no return." Individual may be denying himself pleasure. Stop-start technique is helpful.
Inhibited ejaculation:	may be turned off by vaginal penetration, angry at partner, Also caused by nerve damage.
Dyspareunia: (painful sex)	caused by a tight foreskin that doesn't pull back easily during erection or vascular problems in the penis.

FEMALE DIFFICULTIES	POSSIBLE CAUSE
Lack of arousal:	early trauma, power struggle, anger, boredom.
Dyspareunia	endometriosis, vaginal or pelvic infection, lack of lubrication, anger, tension.
Vaginismus (involuntary tightening of vaginal muscles that makes penetration impossible):	fear of penetration, anxiety, tension. Can be relieved with exercises using fingers or dildo to expand vagina gradually.
Inhibited female orgasm (IFO)	is the inability to achieve orgasm: (30 percent of all women may experience orgasmic problems). Causes may be anxiety, tension, inadequate pleasuring before penetration, lack of manual and oral stimulation of vulva, clitoris and breasts.

There are physical and emotional reasons for all male and female problems, and most of the physical ones can be successfully treated. The mind is another matter. Just because you don't have any organic symptoms doesn't mean you should automatically desire sex and be able to communicate sexually. A person who has suffered incest or abuse in childhood, or who has been traumatized in other ways in his or her relations to the outside world, will find it difficult if not impossible to reach out sexually.

You have to want to heal in order to go and get help. Those who have been turned off to sex for many years, perhaps for an entire adult lifetime, may be in denial about reasons that sex hurts, or that that they have no sex drive. A compassionate partner is a wonderful asset—someone who can bring love to bear when sex isn't wanted. And if you want professional help, it's there for you—psychotherapy and sexual counseling are usually the best resources for couples experiencing any of these painful difficulties.

What About Erectile Dysfunction?

Sexually, the one problem that terrifies men of all ages is what used to be called impotence, but is now termed, *erectile dysfunction.* (They sound equally bad to me, but the first is a clinical term, and I beg forgiveness for sticking it in, so to speak.) Every male individual interviewed for this book at some point mentioned a fear of not being able to get it up, or keep it up, even if he had never experienced the problem.

Is it a big problem? Different sources give widely differing reports. A new federally financed study in Massachusetts claims that nearly half of all American men (about nineteen million) between the ages of forty and seventy experience erectile dysfunction sometimes or all the time. Earlier accounts put the number at ten million. But who's counting when you're personally scared that this dreaded dysfunction may cripple you at some point in your adult life? The more frightened you are that it may happen, the more likely it is to happen, since it's the mind, as we know from Chapter Two, that tells the penis how to behave.

Impotence is defined as the inability to achieve an erection sufficient for penetration and ejaculation 75 percent of the time (during three out of four encounters). This particular condition occurs in 55 percent of men by the time they reach age seventy-five. And even if a man doesn't qualify as clinically impotent, he may have enough difficulty with his erections to warrant seeing a urologist and getting medical or psychological attention.

Why are erections so unreliable? If you are confused as to how erections happen, go back to Chapter Two for a refresher. But let us think about all the various ways and means that a penis might not get hard. There is alcoholism and drug abuse, medications that prevent adequate blood flow to the penis, marital problems, trouble at work, financial woes, children in conflict. There is also a big span of disorders that could have to do with the vascular system (heart, arteries and veins), the endocrine system (radical depletion of testosterone, thyroid condition, diabetes), or the neurologic system (MS, spinal cord injury, epilepsy), the musculoskeletal system (lack of mobility, pain), the respiratory system (chronic obstructive pulmonary disease), and a whole range of emotional illness (anxiety, depression, bereavement and the big catch-all, stress).

Recently, researchers have discovered that a defect in the *nitric oxide* system of the penis can also affect erection. This chemical triggers a chain of events that makes the penis engorge with blood and stay hard. When the system breaks down, the smooth muscles of the penis can't relax—the response that allows the blood vessels in the penis to open and the caverous bodies to fill with blood. In the future, there may be a medication to correct this chemical imbalance.

A variety of tests can be done to see whether erectile problems are psychogenic or physical, and you'll need to see a professional to find out if you warrant such an evaluation. Your family doctor can probably refer you to a urologist who specializes in sexual difficulties. How do you know if your problem is serious? If you can't achieve an erection while masturbating, if you never awaken with an erection or if your penis only gets hard right before ejaculation, it's a good idea to get yourself evaluated.

The urologist will do a complete medical history and perform some blood tests to see whether you might have diabetes or whether your hormonal levels are abnormally low. You'll then be asked to have an NPT (noctural penile tumescence) test.

Any male who is physically capable of achieving and maintaining an erection goes through several cycles each night during sleep where he experiences nocturnal penile tumescence (NPT). It was during these periods in his adolescence when he typically would have had a "wet dream," i.e., when his erection would have reached its logical conclusion in ejaculation. These NPTs occur through the male lifespan into venerable old age, although there are fewer per night as men get older.

And rather than ask a partner to stay up all night watching your penis's ups and downs, you can spend a few nights in a sleep laboratory to check this function. During the test, a device called a RigiScan (yes, really!) is placed around the penis which registers each episode of NPT. It shows how often you're erect, how full the erection is, and how long it lasts. If you're having a few NPTs each night, this means that there is no physiological basis to your erectile dysfunction.

Your physician may also have you tested for penile blood flow in a vascular diagnostic laboratory. The *duplex Doppler exam* will give the doctor a clear picture of your penile arteries; the *cavernosonogram* is an X-ray taken after dye is injected into the penis to follow the pattern of your blood flow.

There is no need to suffer with erectile disorders, or feel humiliated about seeking help. The more silent you are about your concern, the more frequently you will probably find yourself unable to get it up or keep it up. Many men who felt as though they'd been stripped of their masculinity found that changing a medication for hypertension or lowering a dosage of a medication could restore them to complete functionality; others were willing to consider psychotherapy or stress reduction techniques; still others decided that surgery was warranted.

More research is done in this area each year. (Would that there were as many female scientists with a personal stake in the matter to devote such passionate energy to the HRT problem!) There are mechanical, pharmacological and surgical solutions. Not all of these are one hundred percent effective, and not everyone is willing to accept treatments that may be painful or disruptive of the "magic" of sex. However, for a person or couple with a chronic condition, these alternatives should be explored:

- *Vacuum device.* A plastic cylinder is placed over the penis and by pressing a lever, you can pump air out of the cylinder, creating a vacuum which draws blood into the penis and causes it to become erect. You remove the cylinder, placing a specially designed band around the base of the erect penis. It can stay in place for half an hour, but no longer, since it has a tourniquet-like effect. Most men prefer the vacuum pump to giving their penis an injection (see below).

- *Pharmacological therapy (intracorporal injections).* Three different drugs, *papaverine, phentolamine* and *prostaglandin E_1* can be injected into the spongy tissue (the *corpora*) of the penis, causing the arteries and smooth muscles to relax and permit increased blood flow to the area. Within a quarter to half an hour of injecting yourself, you'll have an erection that may last for half an hour to an hour. The treatment is difficult for some men who can't bear the thought of sticking a needle into that particularly vulnerable site. There is some pain involved—from the medication, not the shot. But the therapy does work.

- *Penile Implants (penile prosthesis surgery).* There are several types of surgically implanted aids, either semirigid .or inflatable. The semirigid uses a pair of silicon rods that are placed inside the penis. These bend down against the leg when an erection is not desired. The inflatable implants use hollow cylinders that are placed in the caverous bodies of the penis. These attach to a pump which is squeezed manually for the desired erection.

- *Vascular surgery.* Erections are problematic for men with cardiovascular disease, since it is difficult or impossible to get good blood flow through constricted penile blood vessels. *Revascularization* is a possibility for a man with a normal NPT test who has arterial deficiency. This is called the "penis steal syndrome," since blood that should have flowed into the penis during an erection is "stolen" and rerouted to the thighs. Penile bypass surgery can be performed to correct this condition, but there are certain strict criteria for becoming a candidate—you must be under sixty years of age, not a diabetic or suffering from any neurological disorder.

Venous corporal incompetence is a condition that results from a leaking vein in the corpora. This prevents blood from being properly trapped in the penis, preventing an erection. In order to detect where the leakage occurs, your physician will order a cavernosonogram, or a radiographic X-ray, where a contrast dye is infused into the spongy tissue of the penis. The surgery consists of either ligating or cauterizing the faulty vein.

- *Constriction bands.* These devices were known in the days of the ancient Chinese, and are still useful today. Known in street slang as "cock rings," or "performance rings," these metal or plastic bands are useful for men who can achieve an erection but can't maintain it after penetration. The band is placed around the base of the penis, trapping the blood, and is kept there until after ejaculation.

- *Twenty-first century technology.* In the future, science looks forward to an electrobionic device powered by batteries that might inflate and deflate by a flick of a remote control switch.

But leaving aside the notion of bionic penis power, there's something else to remember about male sexual potential. As Abram, the medical writer of 62 with hypertension said, "I discovered a whole new world of sex when I couldn't rely on my dick all the time. I can't say I'm glad it happened, but it sure did expand my repertoire."

If a medical workup shows no indication of a somatic problem, the next road to take is psychological. The point of sex therapy is to reduce your anxiety about performance and allow you to concentrate on your own pleasure. The exercises in this book and many others (see Resource section) will amplify your therapy.

What About Female Dysfunction?

Women's sexual dysfunction is only coming into its own as an area of exploration and importance in sex therapy. Who ever knew—or cared—whether women were having a comfortable time in bed, let alone, great pleasure? After all, a woman doesn't have to "perform." She can just lie there and pretend everything is hunky dory and no one will know that she's not feeling a thing. Or possibly feeling excruciating pain.

Lack of arousal is the first problem that many women face, and yet there are those who don't acknowledge this as the problem. If they have been abused as children, if they engage in a power struggle in their primary relationship, or if they are simply bored to tears with their partner, they may find other avenues for their sexuality. It is only when such a woman becomes involved with a partner who begins to make some demands about intimacy that she may start to wish to change. A compassionate counselor or sex therapist will recommend graded masturbation and sensate focus exercises for the couple (see Chapter 11).

Inhibited female orgasm (IFO) may occur in fully 30 percent of the female population sometimes or all the time. Is this really a disorder? The reasons are usually a complicated array of factors. I believe the most significant is the woman's insistence that it's her partner's fault. As long as you don't take responsibility yourself, you don't have to do anything to change. But if you really want orgasms, you have to learn to give them to yourself, first, alone as you masturbate, and then with a sensitive partner under the direction of a professional counselor.

There's no way to ignore the other problems of female sexual dysfunction because they hurt so much. *Dyspareunia* is a catch-all term for painful sex, whether it stems from endometriosis, vaginal or pelvic infection, lack of lubrication, or from psychological sources such as anger and tension. Physical sources for pain should be explored with a gynecologist; emotional sources with a therapist or counselor.

Vaginismus, an involuntary tightening of vaginal muscles or persistent vaginal spastic contractions in the muscles at the entrance to the vagina can make penetration impossible. The causes of this disorder are generally terrible fear of penetration or some underlying anxiety or tension around the sexual experience. Although the cause is generally emotional, and the cure must involve some amount of psychological counseling, there are physical tools a woman can use. First, she must learn to touch herself gently and practice exercises using her fingers or a dildo to expand her vagina gradually.

Sex therapy is one answer for women with sexual dysfunction, and it can be helpful whether you have a partner or not. Through directed masturbation, a woman can learn to enjoy herself physically. But no amount of practice makes perfect in the realm of sexual pleasuring, and the body's response is only one part of the puzzle. A great deal of inner exploration and confrontation of serious issues will undoubtedly be essential before a woman who is afraid of sex or has sexual inhibitions will be able to heal successfully.

How to Enjoy Sex Throughout a Chronic Illness

Should sick people have sex? Do they want sex? Of course they *should* if they *do*—physicians feel it is good therapy to feel good and it can be beneficial in terms of flexibility and strength as well. People who loved sex before they got sick will continue to find a way; those who couldn't care less will probably use their illness as an excuse for curtailing activity. Dr. George Ehrlich, adjunct professor of medicine at the University of Pennsylvania, tells the following story: "We had a woman patient who was in the intensive care unit . . . . Yet, while lapsing in and out of coma, she continued to take her birth control pills. When asked about this, she said, 'Well, someday I'm going to be out of ICU and I want to be prepared.'"

One surprising benefit to chronic illness is that it changes your status as a person and that total change invites other changes. A "cancer patient" is no longer seen by her friends and colleagues as a wife, mother, interior decorator, but as someone who is living with cancer. Often, people who are very sick become more open to new possibilities of feeling and behavior. The parameters of touch, whether you're dressed or undressed, whether you make love in the dark or the light, may all be subject to re-evaluation.

Rob was sixty when he had bypass surgery. For at least ten years prior to the event, he'd been on Inderal and several other beta blockers which had wreaked havoc with his sex life.

"I was furious with my body," he said. "It betrayed me. But the angrier I got, the sicker I got. I decided it was too tough, especially in the context of my stable marriage, to explore things with other women that I really wanted to; then after the arteries started going, I couldn't anyway. But my wife and I discovered a whole lot about pleasuring one another when I started falling apart."

But what about the risks? Isn't it too dangerous for a man who's suffered a heart attack or a woman with chronic obstructive pulmonary disease to have an orgasm? Just as with the superstitions surrounding birth and sex, we must break down some old barriers here.

To reaffirm life, we must be able to muster our determination to keep going no matter what. By retaining ties to our sexuality, even when chronically ill, we can make a difference in our healing process. Very few activities in life remind us so keenly of our vitality as this renewal of body and spirit.

*W*HY ILLNESS AND SEX DO MIX

- Sick people are sexual, too. Sometimes their brush with death informs them of just how much they have to celebrate in life.

- Sex after or during an illness may have to be moderated to accommodate the changes in the body and the medications that alter physical reaction. This means both partners must be sensitive to one another's new needs—and old needs.

- It's okay to discuss sex with your physician, but most doctors are not expert in sexual counseling and may be more embarrassed than you about dealing with the subject. If you find you're getting short shrift, there are many professionals who specialize in recuperative sex therapy.

Cardiovascular Disease

Most people who've had a heart attack are terrified of a return to the sexual arena. Yes, there have been instances of overly athletic sex triggering myocardial infarction, but they are few and far between. With your doctor's okay, you can resume sexual activity four to six weeks after a heart attack, and usually the same period of time after heart surgery.

The rule is that if you don't get short of breath, or experience chest pain when you climb two flights of stairs, you can tolerate sex. If you're a man, your heart rate might be 130 on the stairs, and 117 after an exciting bout in bed. If you're a woman, your heart rate might rise as high as 150 at orgasm. Remember though, that this elevation in rate is of very brief duration, and will subside quickly thereafter. A monitored aerobic exercise program as you recuperate will improve your heart's capacity for sex.

Don't have sex after a heavy meal—your heart will direct more blood flow to the stomach to aid in digestion at that time.

Be sure to avoid positions where you're up on your arms a lot. Side-to-side positions tend to be best.

You may feel tired and depressed after you've been ill; your partner may be overprotective and this may bug the hell out of you, making you feel less loving.

If you're having erectile problems or your libido doesn't feel up to snuff, this may have to do with the medications you're on, or the fact that one partner feels a pressure to perform. Speak to your doctor about the effects of these medications and how dosages might be better titrated. Check some of the ideas in Chapter Ten for adding energy and interest to your love life without intercourse.

You should call your physician if you have heart palpitations that last longer than fifteen minutes after sex, or if you're having any difficulty breathing.

Cancer

This ravaging disease brings with it depression and anxiety that can adversely affect the sexuality of any couple. Since cancer is usually such a slow process, it can erode a relationship over time. But it can also work the other way. According to Barbara Rabinowitz, administrative director of the Cancer Center at Monmouth Medical Center, New Jersey, cancer can draw a couple closer and enhance the fiber of their relationship. The reason, of course, is that the couple can really cherish the days they have with one another.

The less the person with cancer is made to feel like a victim, the more sexual he or she can be. Taking charge of where and when love making takes place can be an important step for a person with cancer.

It's easy to worry, illogical as it is, that what you have is "catching" and that you will infect your partner—or that you may have a recurrence of a cancer currently in remission by engaging in sexual activity. These are old myths and have a lot to do with our guilts and fears of pleasure (see Chapter Four).

Anyone who's had radical procedures such as ostomies or who must wear limb prostheses has additional adjustment problems and often worries about turning off their partner (see Chapter Seven). It's crucial for both partners to discuss the fact that they can accept and love one another in a slightly different physical configuration.

Finally, medications can make a big difference in the feeling of both partners. During a course of chemotherapy, it can be too draining and exhausting even to consider being sexual. Then, too, certain chemicals in the therapy have been shown to decrease androgen levels permanently. Androgens are necessary for desire and orgasm. This means that being sensual—exchanging hugs, kisses, and loving touches—becomes more important.

PROSTATE CANCER. This malignancy, a pathological enlargement of the gland just behind the base of the penis, usually affects men over fifty. Self-exams of the testicles and prostate and a rectal exam every year after the age of fifty are crucial preventive-care tactics. All prostate glands enlarge with age, but if urination has become difficult or painful, if there is blood in the urine, or if you are having erection problems, you should see a urologist to check this out. There are many new surgical methods and drugs for this condition, and it certainly need not involve a loss or diminution of your sex life.

One in eleven men currently have prostate cancer; thirty-two thousand men died of it in 1992. If caught early, only the gland itself need be removed; but if it goes undetected and spreads to the lymph nodes and bones, the vas and testicles will have to be removed as well. (The reason for this is that the testes produce testosterone, which helps the cancer to grow.) This is why self-exams are so vital, and all men should do them regularly.

Men who've had a radical prostatectomy can still have erections and enjoy the sensation of ejaculation, although they are no longer fertile.

BREAST CANCER. Probably more women are afraid of dying of breast cancer than of any other illness. It is a specter that hangs over us, whether or not we're at risk. And it's not illogical for us to be concerned, since one in eight women contract breast cancer in America, typically after the age of fifty. Self-exams once a month are essential, as are mammograms every two years, unless you have a family history of estrogen-dependent cancer in which case it should be every year.

Breast cancer wreaks havoc with a woman's self-image (see Chapter Seven), but with a loving partner, and a good period of recuperation, it need not interfere with your sex life. Petra, who had a recurrence of breast cancer four years after her mastectomy, said, "I'm with the business of having this disease every moment, so death is with me all the time. But when Jim and I are together in moments that are so intimately ours, I am alive and concentrated on my aliveness."

If you must have a mastectomy, it will take you time to recuperate physically and even longer emotionally. You will be tired and sore after the surgery and may have difficulty raising your arm or getting into certain positions that require weight on your arms. Side-by-side sex is best until you're completely healed.

Chemotherapy, if required, can drain you of energy, eliminate your sex drive, and cause problems with lubrication. During a course of chemo, you and your partner may wish to concentrate on sensual massage and touch, rather than sex.

HIV/AIDS

Right after an AIDS diagnosis, many couples are overwhelmed. The kind of stress lovers go through at this point may take a toll on their sex life. Many couples choose to be abstinent; but those who don't must use safer sex practices each and every time they make love.

When the PWA (person with AIDS) is healthy, he or she may or may not want to be sexual with a partner, but both desire and response will change considerably over the course of the disease. A person who enjoyed sex prior to AIDS certainly has more chance of enjoying it after infection than a person who didn't particularly care about it before infection. But human sexual response is difficult to chart under the best of circumstances, and when illness strikes, it can take a totally unpredictable course.

When the PWA is struck with various opportunistic infections, he or she may be too weak and exhausted to enjoy sex. This does not mean, however, that he's lost all ability and feeling for physical contact. One of the best things about adjusting your sexual practices around HIV disease is that you both learn new ways of expressing yourselves emotionally and physically. As I've said repeatedly throughout this book, intercourse is not the be-all and end-all of sex, and in fact, other methods of pleasuring one another may be more intimate, last longer, and be just as satisfying to both partners.

When the PWA is very sick and barely able to manage eating, sleeping, and eliminating, it logically follows that sexual activity of any kind will be too taxing and that sexual desire will vanish. This does not mean that you should stop hugging and holding your partner—as a matter of fact, this kind of physical care has been shown to lift spirits and create motivation to go on living.

If you as partner to someone with AIDS are having a lot of difficulty in managing without a full sex life, you may begin to consider other sexual partners. There is nothing wrong with you for feeling this way! The libido in a healthy person is a strong influence. If you are spending twenty-four hours a day with someone who is close to death, you may feel a real need to take comfort from someone healthy. If you should decide to take a sexual partner, understand that this is a serious responsibility. You must, of course, practice safer sex with this other person, but you must also be aware of the potential for hurt, both to your PWA and to this outsider, that exist. This is not to say you can't manage both relationships, but neither will be easy. Of course, nothing about the AIDS experience is easy.

Chronic Obstructive Pulmonary Disease (COPD)

Anyone with chronic bronchitis, asthma, or emphysema will have difficulty breathing and may also experience trouble with motor skills and perception. Sexual arousal may trigger spasms of coughing or bronchial spasms, which may make both partners feel anxious. The terror of suffocation can stop all intimacy dead in its tracks.

Making love at different times of the day when the COPD partner feels freshest and less fatigued can improve both interest and participation in sex. Position is also very important. The partner who has trouble breathing can be propped up on pillows. He or she shouldn't have weight on the chest during sex—a side-by-side position, facing or "spoon"-ing is best. A waterbed, which gives a lovely sexy feel to the whole experience anyway, can be helpful for support and relaxation.

If you have COPD, you know your limits. Always stop what you're doing if you're short of breath. Your partner may want to give you some calming massage as you recover from a spasm.

Men with COPD very often have erectile dysfunction because testosterone levels can be suppressed. If this is your situation, you'll have to talk with your partner about taking a more active role. It's nothing to be ashamed of if you can't be a sexual athlete—you can do less but get more out of it if you learn to relax.

Arthritis/Chronic Pain

Pain and Pleasure

How Pain Works: If you bump your knee, the nerve signals in your knee send messages to the spinal cord and from there to the brain that a painful event has occurred. But not every pain message gets through to the brain because the central nervous system can open and close like a gate to admit or deny entrance to pain stimuli. An athlete in the midst of a fierce football game may have no awareness of a broken rib.

Thoughts and emotions can also change the pain picture. If you feel good, you will have decreased muscle tension, an increase in blood flow to the affected area, and more endorphin production. If a person's thoughts and emotions are bound up in the warmth of a sexual encounter, she may forget the discomfort in another part of her body. Suppose she has pain in her lower back but enjoys lovemaking. Pleasurable sensations in her vagina may take precedence over painful ones in her lower back. The focus of her most impressionable stimulus has shifted from back to vagina.

Historically, pain was often associated with good sex. Gouty pain was supposed to act as an aphrodisiac, and even a life-threatening disease like tuberculosis was given a haze of erotic power by the writer Thomas Mann in his brilliant novel, *The Magic Mountain.*

Pain has always had an interesting connection with pleasure. There are individuals who engage in sexual acts that will specifically cause pain—this is not usually a healthy adaptation to sexuality, but it is more common than we think and not relegated solely to fringe or disturbed couples.

It is probably safest to say that when we are able to get past pain, to open ourselves up to feeling it as opposed to hiding from it or masking it, we can use it to our advantage.

Over thirty-one million individuals (twenty million of them are women) suffer from the crippling, painful rheumatic diseases known collectively as arthritis. Stiffness and limitation of movement in addition to hip pain make sex difficult, and many people who suffer from chronic pain and who are taking strong analgesic drugs may simply not feel interested in sex.

There are many therapeutic avenues to explore if you have arthritis. A program of exercise designed to ease and strengthen muscles—bicycle ergometer and swimming—can improve the potential for sexual activity. Positions, warm baths, and manual aids are enormously important. If it's hard to feel relaxed when in pain, a soak in a tub (with your partner if possible) may set the mood for sexual intimacy. If fingers are too deformed to touch or masturbate effectively, a device such as a vibrator with a special grip can be a real boon.

One form of arthritis suppresses glandular secretions, which means that you may suffer from chronic dry mouth and dry vagina. Lubrication is an absolute must, and should be used at every sexual encounter.

Many arthritis sufferers think that sex will make the pain worse, so they are overly careful with themselves. Actually, studies by Drs. Sadoughi and Brown and others have shown that *people can achieve up to six hours of pain relief after the relaxation and release of sexual activity*. Dr. George Ehrlich, of the University of Pennsylvania, says that the most important thing is to break down barriers with good, honest verbal communication. If your partner thinks he'll hurt you and you interpret this as aversion instead of consideration, you're both in trouble. Talking, however, can bring new levels of sexual intimacy (see Chapter Six).

Headache, another form of chronic pain, is the oldest excuse in the book for avoiding sex. However, certain individuals find great relief after orgasm, possibly due in part to an increased vascular flow in the genital area, away from the head where it usually causes all the trouble.

The biggest sexual problem about having a chronic illness is the erosion of communication between partners that so often occurs. When you feel great, it's easier to express your wants and desires; when you're physically ill most of the time, it can be an insurmountable burden just to ask for your partner's approval and comfort. But if you're to continue being sexual together—and it's good for your emotional health as well as your physical well-being to do so—you've got to open up and talk.

How to Enjoy Sex If You Are Disabled

As discussed in Chapter Seven, our society is hung up on the way the body is supposed to look. If we are different in any way, we are suspect. This is true of every swing away from "the norm," including obesity, congenital abnormalities such as a massive birthmark or deformed limb, scarring from burns or accidents, or any disability.

Why do people talk louder to someone who is blind? Why do they grimace or smile too broadly at someone who is deaf? Why are people in wheelchairs either totally ignored or treated like children? We are simply so uncomfortable looking at or dealing with people who aren't "like us," we can't even handle the most elementary social intercourse. Let alone sexual intercourse!

Getting together intimately with a disabled person is in and of itself considered strange by society's standards. Yet there are thousands of enormously happy "mixed" couples who share their lives, their hopes and dreams, and get undressed and give each other pleasure, like everyone else. There are also mutually disabled couples, who undoubtedly met because of their disabilities, but who discovered a lot more in common than just the fact that they had some functional differences.

Let us get this straight: Disability is *not* disease. And each disability, impairment, or handicap is unique to the person who has it. The World Health Organization defines things this way:

Disability: any restriction or lack of ability to perform an activity in the manner or within the range considered normal for a human being.

Impairment: any loss or abnormality of psychological, physiological, or anatomical structure or function.

Handicap: a disadvantage for a given individual resulting from an impairment or disability that limits or prevents the fulfillment of a role that is normal, depending on age, sex, social and cultural factors for that individual.

The biggest health risk for disabled individuals is not what they can or can't do with their limbs, or how sexual activity may exhaust them or cause them pain. The greatest risk is in their loss of self-esteem and self-worth when they are *desexualized* by society. The intrepid Linda Crabtree, a Canadian sex educator, published an amazing story in her newsletter, "It's Okay!" a wonderful publication about sexuality and disability.

The writer of the article, a woman in a wheelchair from a childhood bout with polio, had switched places with her able-bodied boyfriend before the bar filled up. She was sitting on a barstool, and he sat in her wheelchair for the evening. Men flirted with her, offered to buy her drinks, treated her as they would any other available woman. They patted her male friend on the back as he sat, supposedly helpless, supposedly sexless, and, therefore, not a male worth competing with.

Women ignored him or patronized him, wiping out any possibility for him to make a connection—however innocent—with any of them. The final insult: The bartender questioned him about his tolerance for alcohol, implying that he didn't know his own limit and couldn't control himself if he went past it. (Surely no able-bodied male would want to have to help him in the men's room should there be an emergency.)

If we can get past the thinking, then there are just two bodies, two people, just like any others. But that is a very tall order indeed.

Some particular conditions that may or may not affect the ease of a sexual relationship are:

- Spinal cord injuries (paraplegia or quadriplegia which cause partial or total paralysis)
- Polio and postpolio syndrome (lack of use but not feeling in legs and possible breathing difficulties requiring a respirator)
- Multiple sclerosis (periods of partial paralysis and numbness, tingling, changes in sensory perception)
- Muscular dystrophy and other neuromuscular diseases (progressive weakening and degeneration of the muscles)
- Cerebral palsy (lack of muscle coordination, spastic movements, tremors, difficulty with speech)
- Blindness
- Deafness
- Epilepsy
- Endocrine disorders (dwarfism or gigantism)
- Amputation

What is different about sex for people who are disabled? In some cases, lots, and in some cases, not much at all. The concerns fall into the following areas:

- Meeting people with whom you might want to have an intimate relationship
- Getting past "the dreaded chair syndrome"
- Difficulty breathing
- Motility, positions, restriction of movement
- Cleanliness and hygiene
- Difficulty managing spastic bladder/placement of the catheter
- Lack of ability to have an erection and/or ejaculation

None of these issues will prevent a disabled person from wanting to be sexual or being sexual. Some have the capacity for physical orgasm; others may not, but their brain will supply the needed enhancement for an erotic experience to be just as satisfying. Many women who have no use of their hands or are paralyzed and cannot move report being able to have orgasms through visualization only. New erogenous zones develop when others are knocked out, so nipples may become as sensitive as a clitoris used to be, depending on the location of the injury. Luckily, because the human mind and body is so flexible, even when injured or disabled, there are options:

- Vibrators are useful to achieve and maintain an erection in the man and to sufficiently arouse a woman so that she can lubricate.
- Water-based lubricants are useful for both partners, both to avoid irritation and to increase sensitivity, and because they're fun.
- A man with a spinal cord injury can be manually stimulated to get an erection. If the erection isn't sufficient for penetration, he or his partner can use the "stuffing" technique—placing the penis inside the vagina so that she can grip with her PC muscles.
- A stretchable tape or cock ring can be placed around the base of the penis to keep it engorged until penetration is achieved.
- Since bowel and bladder control may be difficult, both partners should be sure to go to the bathroom prior to sexual activity. External catheters and leg bags can be removed; indwelling catheters shouldn't cause any problem as long as there's sufficient lubrication.

And if there's no partner at the moment, just as with ABs (able-bodied persons), there is always masturbation. Even without use of the hands, there are a variety of implements, home-made and purchased, to assist in self-loving. See the Resource Guide at the back of this book for particular information.

Sexual adjustment is only one small piece of the puzzle for disabled people. We next approach the loaded issue of who they're supposed to be sexual with. Our society tends to make nonable-bodied individuals feel that if they are entitled to love at all, that it should be with one of their own kind. But what a cruel way to segregate feelings! In many cases, people who were injured feel cheated—they were once "normal," having the same chances for love as everyone else—and suddenly they were in a different category. A lot of suppressed anger often surfaces in a person who feels it would be "settling" to fall in love with or marry another similarly disadvantaged person.

For those born with a particular condition or impairment, they too often grow up with a lasting impression of how unwanted they are. Luckily, there are those who can be color-blind, height-blind, impairment-blind. It is to the credit of all disabled people who are able to cherish and love themselves enough to love another, like or unlike them.

Guidelines for Healthy Sexual Choices

Sex is so personal, so special to each of us that the distinction between what's right and wrong about it really can't be dictated by anyone standing outside your relationship. When you feel you need to make a decision, don't examine your criteria against anything other than the following:

- Do we both want to?
- Will this hurt us or anyone else?
- Are there ways we can express ourselves that aren't sexual that will further the relationship right now?

Talk to yourself, talk to your partner, and then decide. If you aren't "right" one hundred percent of the time, be forgiving and don't aim for such a high score.

10

How
to Increase
Your Sexual
Energy

*S*ex is not your average health-oriented activity. It is not like running a mile or swimming a few laps. It bears little in common with skiing (except for that moment of delight and thrill when you feel yourself whizzing downhill too fast), and it bears no resemblance to tennis.

It does, however, require the same or more energy, and for some people who aren't in great shape, the very physical elements combined with the emotional rush can be taxing.

To make your sex life exciting, you have to be exciting. This may require some work on your part. You don't want to be huffing as you chase your paramour up the stairs; you don't want to give out after an hour of strenuous lovemaking. Even multiple orgasms can knock you out if you're not prepared for them.

*E*XPERT-LEVEL SEXUALITY

Celia, a graduate student who was recently divorced, decided after a course in human sexuality that she could top the one hundred orgasms experienced by a woman masturbating from the example in her textbook. One snowy afternoon, she tried to beat the record, just for fun. She told me she had counted sixty-five when the doorbell rang. Limp and panting, she crawled to the door but couldn't get up to open it. Her friend from down the block demanded through the closed door that she get off her duff and come out to throw snowballs with him. She politely demurred, saying she was otherwise occupied. Celia didn't walk straight for the next three days. But she felt wonderful.

Exercises That Will Spark Your Sex Life

It is now a matter of documented record that regular exercise prevents disease, helps us to maintain body weight, raises our endorphins (the natural opiates in the brain that make us feel good), and may prolong life just a little as well.

It is also documented that people who feel fit have better sex lives. Over a nine month period, a group of sedentary men were asked to participate in a daily aerobic program. They were asked to keep a diary about their sexual performance and interest. The seventy-eight participants found that their interest in sex, their performance, the nature of their orgasms and their frequency of different intimate activities were all enhanced by their improved fitness. Those who had described themselves as having a low sex drive found that their libidos increased. They fantasized more, masturbated more, and had intercourse more.

The men who stopped smoking in addition to exercising even had greater sexual benefits—they experienced more orgasms, and they were more fulfilling. All the men also reported that they felt less anxious after the program. Whether this was because they were in better physical health or because their sex lives had improved was not determined.

Let's look at this clinically for a moment.

- Exercise lowers LDL cholesterol, which tends to narrow arteries by allowing plaque to build up.

- An erection takes place because blood flows freely through the vessels leading to the penis. Atherosclerotic changes in the arteries supplying blood to the penis make for increased erectile problems. But lower LDLs improve the dilation of these vessels.

- Torquing the body during sex is easier when your joints are flexible.

- Orgasmic pleasure may increase with better internal and external muscle tone.

- Intense short-term exercise seems to increase men's testosterone level, possibly because of hormonal changes in the concentration of androgens in the blood during the exercise period.

- There is some evidence that there may be a correlation between increased brain endorphins and enhanced sexuality—possibly because feeling good and relaxed is a prerequisite for being orgasmic. Increased melatonin, the neurotransmitter produced by the pineal gland that makes us feel relaxed and sleepy, is another benefit of increased exercise.

Of course, lest you all go out and start Olympic training to become sexual athletes, I must point out that *too* much exercise dampens the sexual response. Low testosterone levels in marathoners is common—which lowers their libidos and may even depress their beard growth. Women who overtrain may stop ovulating and menstruating—their hormonal system shuts down to protect their body from what the brain perceives as a state of acute physical stress. And if they're not menstruating, these women may start to worry about their reproductive abilities—which in turn can take away their desire for sex. Although some women may feel more at ease because of a lowered risk of pregnancy, others may feel less feminine and therefore, inadequate to the challenge of sexual desire.

Other studies indicate that runners tend to get divorced more than other people, and that male runners, in particular, cheat on their wives more. Does this prove anything about their sexuality? Maybe runners, typically Type A individuals, are rarely satisfied with anything, from the time it takes them to sprint a half-mile to their marriages.

---

*W*ORK-OUT FOR THE BEDROOM

To be in really good physical shape for lovemaking, it's a good idea to stretch those areas that tend to get used in bed and nowhere else. It is never more disheartening to wake up the morning after a delightful long night and find that you're sore, inside and out.

Here are some easy stretches you can do together, or when you're alone and waiting for your lover. *Don't bounce* into these stretches—it is far more beneficial to pull yourself to

(continued on page 202)

the extent of your stretch, hold it, then breathe and get down
a little further.

- *V-stretches:* Sit on the floor and spread your legs. Pull yourself gently to one leg, then the other, finally to the middle.

- *Cross-stretches:* Sit on the floor and spread your legs. Cross
  one leg over the top of the other and try to touch it with
  your opposite hand. Reverse.

- *Back-stretches:* Sit on the floor, one leg extended in front of
  you, one bent at the knee and tucked behind you. Lean back
  as far as you can go toward your back foot, stretching the
  front of your thigh. Switch legs and reverse.

- *Kegels:* For the inside muscular control you need, both men
  and women should perform pubococcygeal contractions,
  whenever and wherever they can (see Chapter Eight).

What's the best part of exercise as it relates to sex? Sticking to
an exercise program tends to make people feel good about themselves. You prove to yourself that you have the discipline to stay with
a regimen, and your body thanks you by responding and looking
well. One man interviewed for this book talked about his well-toned,
always fit body as though it were a good friend: "I took it out for
walks, gave it showers, provided it with lots of good sex, and in
return, it treated me well."

Couch potatoes tend to see themselves as sloppy, overweight,
depressed, too tired to do much of anything.

Fanatic exercisers are hard on themselves and others, moody,
anxious about weight changes, and very often brusque and cold in
their sexual dealings with others.

Moderate exercisers find that a brisk two-mile walk once a day
every day is sufficient to make them feel wonderful in this corpore-
al house they live in, eager to share it with others.

How to Eat Well for a Better Sex Life

You are what you eat. And consuming a healthy diet can give
you the spark you need to feel comfortable in bed as well as out of
it. Since we are not talking here about sleeping in bed, but being

physically active, it's important that you eat as though you were thinking about exercising afterward.

Big heavy meals are not on for sex. A thick steak, marbled with fat, accompanied by fried potatoes and a milk shake is probably the worst thing you could think about before an amorous encounter. A salad and some fruit, or a nice vegetarian pasta dish is ideal. The idea is to be satiated (and that way your stomach doesn't rumble), not to feel too filled up; you want to be light but strong when you're making love.

And you really want to enjoy this body you are sharing with someone else. As we learned in Chapter Seven, body image has dealt a crippling blow to many in our society. If you always feel fat, you never want to take off your clothes before a mirror or your lover or even your cat. If you like the way your body looks, you are comfortable offering its bounty to someone else. And you shouldn't be monitoring everything you put in your mouth in order to enjoy your body.

Eating well will definitely boost your self-esteem. *Good eating and attitudes toward food* promote sanity at the table and in life, and at the same time, the nutrients you ingest support the structure that holds you together and give you the energy you need for an active sex life.

Poor eating and attitudes toward food make you obsessive and fixated on some idealized notion of how to be something you're not. It detracts greatly from your sense of well-being, and certainly alienates you from a partner who might like to lick hollandaise sauce off you in bed.

Good Eating	Poor Eating
eating a little of everything	junk food
low-fat foods	eating on the run
low-protein foods	irregular meals
low-salt and -sugar foods	yo-yo dieting
high-fiber foods	bingeing
high-carbohydrate foods	purging
eating several small balanced meals a day	

Food can be a great aphrodisiac. The classic scene in the movie *Tom Jones* shows a couple hungry for each other, devouring each other with their eyes, eating this incredible banquet as though they were tucking into one another's flesh. It is funny and sexy at the same time because it parallels one appetite with another. Most of us have experienced the flow of saliva as we regard a mouth-watering meal; and many of us have had that insatiable desire to take a bite out of a lover.

Here's an exercise to try with your partner:

Salt: Share a potato chip; then lick each other's skin.

Sweet: Share an ice cream cone; then kiss.

Sour: Share a pickle; run a lemon along your partner's leg and lick up the length of it.

Bitter: Share a small salad of arugula or chickory; pour a little black coffee at room temperature into the hollow of your partner's throat and drink it.

Examine the different tastes of each other. Your natural juices, of course, are the most distinct flavors, if you enjoy oral sex. Men's ejaculate and women's cum taste different depending on diet and time of the month, and stress can play a factor as well. It is said that vegetarians have sweeter natural secretions and smells.

A Bedroom Feast

The different parts of the body taste different as well, and you can energize your sex life together by making a banquet of your lover. Use the tip of your tongue, the flat of your tongue, your teeth—gently—your whole mouth and plenty of saliva to get a real taste. You may wish to take a bath or shower together first, but don't use any scented soaps, powders or lotions.

You can spread different foods on your lover for this gustatory tour (see Chapter Eleven for a list) or have him or her *au naturel*: toes, in between toes, legs with and without hair, the knob and the back of the knee, the thigh and the inside of the thigh, the scrotum or vulva, the buttocks, the small of the back, the top of the back and the shoulder blades, the upper arms, armpits, elbows, forearms, wrists, hands and fingers, the belly, breasts, clavicles, neck, ears, nose, mouth (at last!), eyes and brows, forehead, scalp, hair. *Bon appetit!*

Flirting: Clever Ways to Recharge Your Sexual Batteries

The French, who are reputed to know more about sex than any other people on earth, have a wonderful expression for flirting. *Rouler les hommes* means to mystify or pull the wool over the eyes of a man. The word *rouler* literally means turn or roll around. Imagine, then, rolling a lover around in your fingers, getting the sense of him, the feel of his body. The expression itself connotes conning or duping, but in the nicest sense. When you flirt, if you do it right, the other person knows it's not really serious—you don't necessarily intend to jump into bed after bantering lightly with each other. Or maybe you do. Who knows?

Flirting exploits the really sexy organ—the brain. When your partner sneaks up behind you and tells you that you smell good enough to eat, you suddenly imagine the two of you in the throes of oral sex. It's wonderful because your mind has no limits, no set number of orgasms. You can allow the flirtation to become one more intimate thing you share.

In today's politically correct environment, however, flirting can be very dangerous. The slightest evidence that the flirter is interested and the flirtee is not can provoke a lawsuit. Sexual harassment is legally defined as "unwanted, unwelcomed sexual behavior that interferes with your life." Some individuals (those, in my opinion, who totally lack a sense of humor and style) think that any flirting is disrespectful of another's privacy and should be banned. So watch your back and watch your mouth before you tread into this hazy arena.

If you go by Webster's definition, you should be in safe territory, but only if you carry a dictionary and can read the following to your partner. "To flirt" is defined as "to play at courtship," and in fact, this is using your sexuality at its best. Play is the key word—I always think the best sex is playful—and too many people take the whole thing too seriously. When you get serious, you get dull. Flirting keeps the edge on a conversation, and in fact, can make some people rather brilliant. Flirting might go like this:

Pass One: Should I wear a skirt tomorrow night?

Pass Two: As long as you don't wear anything underneath it.

Or like this:

Pass One: Gee, it's hot out.

Pass Two: It's hot wherever you are.

Pass Three: Just when you're around. You're the flint to my match.

Pass Four: You're the cream in my coffee. And speaking of cream . . . (speaker looks down meaningfully at lower half of body).

Flirting is a turn-on because it requires concentration and effectiveness. Like "dissing," the rapier-quick ghetto-speak that downgrades others, flirting keeps you on your toes. You have to have a comeback ready, but you can't prepare it. It has to be spontaneous and clever and relevant to the other person.

There is flattery involved in flirting, but mostly, it's implied. It's just plain dumb in this day and age to try to get someone's attention by telling them they're the greatest thing since sliced bread, or that the stars come out when they smile. Lines, like old jokes, are usually too corny to work on anyone who's had a moderate amount of experience with sexual badinage. On the other hand, if somebody tells you that short shorts must have been invented so you could wear them, that's a pretty good ego-boost. It's also flirting because it's a joke as well.

Flirting isn't just verbal, of course. There's a whole gamut of facial expression, raised eyebrows, licked lips, intense stares, and occasionally, warm touches that go along with the banter. The quality of the body language often helps determine where the flirting goes.

Both partners must understand the meaning of the flirting. In a business setting, or at school, for example, this kind of wordplay and physical jostling should stop when work or study starts up again. In an intimate setting, where two friends are getting to know one another, it can go either way.

Flirting can be extremely manipulative. One woman I interviewed told me she consciously used her sexuality when she drove a pickup truck during her summer job. "I'd be the only woman climbing down from a rig when I parked at a truck stop. And if I was having trouble with anything—from the engine to the rear-view mirror, these guys would offer to help me out. I can't explain it, but I really attracted them, and I felt completely safe doing it. I just turned on this different voice and style. Not wimpy or little-girl-helpless at all, but kind of like a sexual sorcerer. Almost like I got bigger, more noticeable, and they would do anything for me. This was certainly flirting, although I never consciously came across as batting my eyelashes. I really hate that—it's a cartoon of sex."

As the prelude to sex or as a recharging of your batteries, flirting stimulates both parties. It's a safe activity as long as it's understood between you what the intention of the flirting is.

Always remember that the teasing and cute remarks, the almost accidental bumping and touching can be misinterpreted. And if it gets out of hand, if you sense that the meaning of the flirting has undergone a sea change while you weren't paying attention, stop and talk it out. It's possible that the other person wants it to lead to a sexual encounter—or that you do, and your partner is playing dumb—or hard to get.

In that case, you'll need a transition from being funny and adorable to being down to earth. Then you'll need to check and see if the other person is following along with you.

How to Get Turned On

Desire is a complex and wonderful feeling. We may spot one body part—a hand, a breast, a butt—that suddenly gives us that rush of longing. We may exchange a glance with a longtime partner across a crowded room and immediately feel desperate to get them alone. We may sit over a cup of coffee with a good friend and be bowled over by a jolt of sexual feeling we never had for this person before. It can happen anywhere, anytime.

Desire is like appetite—you feel hungry for another person. You can lust after them, or after just the sight of their knee. Healthy desire helps us to pick our relationships. We don't always choose the smartest, the most attractive, or the kindest person to have a sexual relationship with. We don't always choose the person who will be the best bet in the long run.

Very often, we want what we can't have. Many people leap from one inappropriate relationship to another, enjoying the fact that their partner is basically unavailable. It is a common turn-on, because ultimately this type of desire requires no great emotional commitment.

The power of desire is enormous, and when it takes over the mind, it can become obsessive. Many people interviewed for the book admitted to having "crushes" on people that led them to make special detours to their house, send them presents, make phone calls (even if they hung up without speaking to the object of their desire). Some individuals have moved across country, given up jobs and taken new ones, changed their entire life to be near a loved one.

If the love is not reciprocated, and the desire is unquenchable, this can lead to severe mental disorders. "Stalking," or following a person against their will, has been much in the news lately. Indeed, there have been those driven to murder and suicide in the name of this type of addictive passion.

Then there's the opposite end of the spectrum—lack of desire. Couples who feel little or no passion for one another may end up together anyway. Unfortunately, this missing element may cause terrible dissatisfaction. Without the kind of erotic stimulus that makes a long partnership constantly exciting, it's hard to retain those other essential feelings like love, respect, and loyalty.

This is not to say that if you don't feel the itch, this is someone to ditch. There may be dozens of other reasons to link up with someone, and in truly close intimate partnerships, desire can grow over time. The heights of sex that we can experience at twenty may be nothing in comparison to the depths of passion we can know at fifty.

It is a fact, however, that some people are never walloped with this dynamic emotion, and many individuals end up in sexual counseling because of "inhibited sexual desire." Of course, you can *have sex* without wanting it much, but this means that your partner must initiate it all the time. And this can lead to real struggles for power in the relationship. Why do you always let me do the work? one partner might ask another. And eventually, if the pursuit is too much work, the initiator might just stop trying.

Desire isn't logical—it works like instinct to fulfill a need. If more of us were able to separate love and sex, there would be less confusion when we desired a person with whom we could never spend the rest of our lives. We could express passion as fully as we wanted with one partner and express strong, nurturing, bonding warmth with another.

But if we combine those feelings of desire and warmth, we can have a truly volatile combination. There is only one way to get turned on, and that is, oddly enough, *not* to rely on our partner to do it. If you are not feeling as much as you want to, it's your job to project some of your fantasies onto the person you are currently involved with. You may be surprised at the results.

How to Turn Yourself On

Use the elements that you think of as "sexy" to change what might be a boring, banal situation. If hot and steamy weather turns you on, put that in the mix; if you like to be bundled in quilts watching the snow come down, add that. Think about clothing—dress your partner (or undress your partner) in the way that reveals his or her body's secrets best. Add the setting: Do you feel more stimulated on a desert island, a crowded street, a mountain chalet, a boarded-up old barn? Add a hint of danger: maybe you're alone in a subway car in New York City with the action of the train throwing you together.

Once you have your "stage" set, put your partner in it. Concentrate on one part of her or him—the eyes, the hands, the buttocks, the breasts—that are most exciting to you. Feel as though that part is projecting itself out of your partner just for you. Let the rest of the body come to you gradually, as though you were examining it for the first time. Add the emotion to it—what is it about this person that draws you together if it's not sex?

Enjoy yourself slowly, quickly, as the initiator and as the recipient of attention. Don't focus on the genitals at all in this exercise—spend the time to find out what it is that you may never have considered about your partner that matches your most erotic desire.

How to Use Fantasy to Trigger and Mold Desire

"When I was in college, in the sixties," Dorie, a forty-nine-year-old copywriter told me, "I was with this group of kids who were all very introspective, very aware. We got together for a party at the end of the school year that turned into an experiment with group sex—

it was really an orgy, in the days when that wasn't completely unsafe. I never thought of myself as somebody who could get turned on by lots of bodies doing it, but my mind went nuts, just seeing these penises and breasts and combinations of male and female.

"I had a pal with me—he and I stayed together for most of it so I didn't feel so exposed—but the night really changed me in some deep way. Before, I'd had this iron thing around sex, like a band that was welded shut around me. But the party broke the band, and it was easier, afterward, to do things and get wrapped up in them. What I wanted and dreamed of could be real."

Hannah, who came out as a lesbian after two marriages, said that a formative sexual experience for her was being shown a training film in a human sexuality course that projected many different sexual scenes at the same time on a big screen. "There were people and animals—I think there were even two elephants doing it! Just watching it, I had an orgasm, not touching myself or anything. The feelings this movie triggered in me were overwhelming, all-encompassing, like my mind was part of all the sexuality of all these beings."

Fantasy, according to Robert May in his book, *Sex and Fantasy*, is "the rich and varied theater that plays in our heads all the time. Scenes of hope and fear, incidents of anger or of lust, retroactive rewritings of history, and tender anticipations of the future—all these are part of the constant buzzing and scuttling that goes on in the darkened backstage area of our mind."

There are thoughts or daydreams floating around in all of us that we wouldn't consider acting on. One man interviewed for this book said he would love to have the opportunity to make love as a woman—although he has no interest whatsoever in real life to be a different gender. Several couples told me they fantasized about having a third person in bed with them (the most common combination being a man and two women), yet only one of the people I spoke to had ever acted on that. Rape fantasies, romantic desert island dreams, group sex—all are in the lexicon of *normal* human interest. We make up these little scenes for ourselves, either during a slow time in the day or while we masturbate, and act them out mentally.

How often do most people fantasize? The frequency ranges from never to several times a day—that is, the long theater pieces that we write in our brain are different from the passing thoughts about sex that flicker through our heads constantly. Several studies have shown that sexual fantasies can help women who are not easily orgasmic reach a climax during intercourse.

Share your fantasies with your partner. If you do, you can really let your imagination fly. Here you must tread carefully, because one member of a couple can be hurt by another's whim. You should know your partner really well before you share a fantasy that may have upsetting elements—from forced sex to sex with many partners, to sex with a stranger to sex with inanimate objects, to bondage, to sex with others watching. But the right mix of elements, told in a comfortable setting, with both individuals as willing participants, can enhance a relationship.

Here are some ways to get started:

1. Rent a pornographic video. Each of you describe one scene to the other that turned you on. Embellish it with your own idea of what you would do with your partner in this situation.

2. Read each other a section of some exciting pornographic literature, such as Anais Nin's *Delta of Venus: Erotica*, or Nancy Friday's *My Secret Garden*. You may want to act out some of the descriptions from the page, or let the events motivate you to think up some creative activities of your own.

3. Tell each other stories, just as you might make up a bedtime story for a child, but with X-rated content. Let your imagination run wild. You may be the hero or heroine, or you may pick anonymous characters. (This is a "safe" way to tell some of your actual fantasies, by couching them in fiction.)

4. Tell each other some of your dreams. Dreams, unlike fantasies, stem from our subconscious awareness, and events don't have to be logical or consecutive. The content of most people's dreams is extremely sexual—we allow ourselves images and acts in our dream life that we would never permit ourselves while awake. Explore these erotic facets in detail with your partner—it will tell you a great deal about yourself and your relationship.

5. Share fantasies. Be considerate of how much and what kind of information your partner can take. Remember that you may not be turned on by the same things. That's okay—it can be fun to be a player in someone else's fantasy. You may get hot and bothered from the idea of making love blindfolded and your partner may react in a similar way to hearing you talk dirty.

Abandon Guilt and Increase Pleasure

If you want to enhance your sexuality and your experience of sex with another person, you must heal from the moral burdens of the past that severely restrict your progress. Many individuals who want to feel free and liberated sexually are saddled with expectations and obligations that stem from long-ago guilt. You may want to experience what it would feel like to be tied to the bed with scarves, but never suggest it for fear your partner might laugh at you. You may have a keen desire to have an erotic phone conversation with your partner when you can't be together, and yet feel as though you're doing something wrong if you say the words out loud.

To abandon guilt, you must decide that what you are doing in the present moment is more important than what others think of you, or what you have thought of yourself in the past. The useful thing about guilt is that combatting it, and doing something that initially makes you feel pretty wicked, can be very exciting.

To get more energy into your sex life, try the following activities:

- *Have phone sex* with someone when they aren't in a position to respond to you even if you feel lewd and lascivious speaking your inmost thoughts.

- *Wear a costume* for your partner—perhaps a garterbelt and bustier if you're a woman; maybe a pair of leather pants with zippers if you're either sex, and let your partner take your clothes off.

- *Undress and dance suggestively* in front of your partner, even if this makes you feel self-conscious about your body and how it moves when you're aroused.

- *Have sex in a semipublic place*—the back of a movie theater or on a blanket at the beach—even if it makes you feel vulnerable to the censure of others.

- *Make love with the lights on* even if you feel uncomfortable because everything, from your excitement to your boredom—can be seen by your partner.

- *Tell your lover what you want and don't want,* even if you feel awkward because it makes you feel greedy, like you're asking for something you don't deserve.

Eleven Ways to Add Vitality and Spontaneity to Your Relationship

Alice and her lover had great difficulty finding places to be intimate. They had decided that it was a mistake to use their own homes for sexual encounters, since they wanted to keep their affair separate from their marriages.

"We hung out in my car a lot," Alice told me, "and explored parking lots, woods, anywhere relatively secluded. There was something so exciting about driving—we didn't know where—thinking what would happen when we parked. Sometimes it was hard to carry on a regular conversation, we were so attracted, so into each other. The car was like our cocoon. When we were inside, nothing could touch us.

"Once we took a picnic—some good red wine that we slugged, passing the bottle back and forth, and a hunk of cheese we cut with my Swiss army knife and ate with grapes and bread. We never took off all our clothes—partly because we never knew if the place was really private, partly because it was pretty cold in those woods. But we had to be contortionists, using our bodies in different ways in such a cramped space. We got good at reading each other's pleasure, riding the waves of getting aroused, then stopping and maneuvering into a new position to keep it going longer. And it was funny, the two of us falling off the seat, bumping our heads, accidentally turning on the overhead light with a random foot in the air—we'd laugh at how ridiculous the whole thing would seem to an outsider.

"It made me more spontaneous with my husband, I think. Even though we had room to take off clothes and lie down in a nice comfortable bed, I'd tend to drag him down on the floor occasionally, which he liked because it told him I wanted him so badly, I couldn't wait."

There is such variety when it comes to playing with the body! All you have to do is change one element and you open up a whole set of doors. The restricted space that Alice and her lover had to work with made them creative. You can try as many different positions as the Kama Sutra recommends, but the best way to enhance your energy in sex is to develop exciting possibilities that arise from natural circumstances.

Space. Try making love using lots of space, then very little. See what you can do in a huge open field and in a dark closet.

Time. Give yourself several hours together to explore each other and your own sensuality. Next time, have a quickie.

No hands. Do everything to one another with mouths, bodies, and feet. See how your other body parts become extra hands. You can give a massage, for example, by rubbing your own torso or buttocks along the length of your partner's back and legs.

Don't look. Try making love blindfolded. First, allow one partner to see and the other to be blindfolded. Then switch roles. Finally, you should both cover your eyes. The anticipation and delicious surprise of what can happen between you is heightened when you don't see what's coming and don't even know what body part or orifice you're touching right away. The two of you may be much more spontaneous about what you do when you can't see.

Talk it out. Tell each other exactly what you want to do before you do it. Choose your words carefully, so that they convey the most sensual meaning possible.

Be silent. Don't say a word or make a sound. You might pretend you're undercover and the least whisper would give you away. As much as you might want to let go and scream when you climax, prevent yourself—and let your partner help—from so much as breathing hard. It's difficult!

Uncommon orifices. You have so many places, crevices, spaces, and nooks you never really use sexually. You could tuck a penis between breasts, armpits, backs of knees or in the crease of the butt, for example. You could put your partner's toes in your mouth and suck each one as though it were a little penis. You could use a knuckle, knee or elbow around and on the vulva. Look at the fabulous architecture of the body—see what each part can really do. Abandon (temporarily!) the comfortable placement of penis in vagina if you're a man and a woman or penis in anus if you're two men and try out the dozens of other possibilities.

In the old days, when people were used to extreme formality in everyday life, it was not expected that touching, holding, kissing, and intercourse would take place within the first few weeks or months of a relationship. But because couples were just as horny then as they are now, they found other means of keeping an edge on the hot and heavy interest.

To enhance the vitality of your own sexuality, you can resurrect some of the older, tried but true courtship tactics:

- Go dancing.
- Spend an afternoon taking tea together.
- Select small gifts for one another that reflect something about your relationship—flowers beautifully arranged, special stationery, a particular piece of music.
- Create a ritual that is all your own and means something significant to the two of you. This may involve making a private space where you can meditate together, finding a hidden place in a park where you can sit and watch the sun come up or go down, or lighting candles and holding hands.

Spontaneity also means going with the moment. Don't plan so much in advance for everything you want to do together—let your excitement move you.

How to Stimulate Your Senses

If you keep in mind that your sexual energy is in great part sensually stimulated, you will never be at a loss for new ways to excite your partner and yourself. In the next century, as we evolve to become more enlightened sexual beings, we may be able to abandon the cult of penis and vagina and concentrate on the five—or six—senses.

Make love

- so that it heightens your sense of *touch*. Make a bed of pillows, so that you are surrounded and held by something soft as you hold each other.
- so that it heightens your sense of *sight*. Surround yourself with color and wear different colors. Select cool colors one time, hot colors another. See what differences this makes in your mood and the way you perceive your partner.
- so that it heightens your sense of *taste*. Try the bedroom feast recommended at the beginning of this chapter and use the foods I suggest in Chapter Eleven. If you practice oral sex

together, consciously change your diet for a week (try heavy on vegetables one week, heavy on fruit the next, heavy on grains and legumes the third week) and see if there is any difference in the taste of your lover.

- so that it heightens your sense of *sound*. Use different music— classical, jazz, blues, rock, and so on—and see how this affects your lovemaking.

- so that it affects your *intuition*, which has been called the sixth sense. Try to read your partner's mind and guess just what he or she is ready for. Open your minds to allow your thoughts to penetrate each other.

- so that it heightens your *life force*. Use breathing consciously together as a means of getting closer. Let one person lead and the other follow in different patterns of breath intake and output and holding—then switch. Visualize moving the breath from your center to your partner's center, down to the sexual organs, then around the perineum and up the back all the way to the top of the head. Feel the sexual energy transmogrify into spiritual energy.

- so that it heightens your *imagination*. Your fantasies and shared visualization can take you both on an unforgettable voyage in sexual awareness. If you open yourselves to the feelings triggered by touch, massage, arousal, and orgasm, you may suddenly find that you've been shortchanging yourself sexually for years and that only now can you appreciate how much more awake and aware you are.

By allowing mind, body, and spirit to take their course, you will gain immeasurably as a sexual being. You will hone the skills you need to be a better lover—to yourself as well as the person with whom you share passion.

11

How
to Make
Love

*A*t last! The chapter you've been waiting for (or, if you're *that* kind of reader, the one you skipped ahead to dip into first).

But the point, of course, is that the healing power you've learned to use throughout this book has already taught you how to make love. You know now that it's very simple and very complicated at the same time. Because making love isn't always the path to ecstasy—it can simply be a way of sharing quiet time, or of relieving tension, or of getting through the night. It can be banal, routine, painful—or it can, every once in a wonderful while, really hit the heights.

We are all flying blind when it comes to making love—there are dozens of manuals instructing us carefully to put a hand here and a mouth there, but the process is different for everyone, and comes out different every single time. We may get ideas from books and movies, we may compare notes with a friend, but we really learn how to make love from our imaginations and cooperative partners.

Basic rules apply:

1. Be kind to yourself.

2. Be kind to your partner.

3. Let your whole body smile.

4. Try not to do anything the same way twice.

5. Don't think so much.

6. Let your body and feelings guide you.

7. Play. Have fun.

How to Develop Your Own Sexual Style

Bill told me about how his energy had grown over the years and changed with his various partners. "I get turned on and turn someone else on because our brains collide. Sure, it's nice to think your body and his is appealing—but that's not what makes me want to make love. Sometimes, I get talking to my lover and then I can't keep my hands off him. I try to incite sex, you know, and it usually works. The thought and action together—it's very powerful for me. When we actually get into it, I may be alternately gentle and forceful, but my style is definitely moving the action."

Dorie said she thought she and her lover always had a mutual knowledge that they wanted to make love. "We'll be standing in the kitchen together, joking around, and the joking will turn into fantasies and what we'd like to do to each other. We kind of talk it out first. Then one of us will say what we want and we'll be holding each other or kissing. I see my way of making love as a part of being a couple—the process of knowing each other so well that the impetus to come together is pretty spontaneous."

Peter said that he and his wife were pretty matter-of-fact in their style. "I'm usually more aware than she is that we both want to make love. I'll just say, 'How about a date?' or 'Do you have any time to go upstairs with me?' I don't like playing around, I come right to the point, and I'm that way physically, too. I move right in and have my hands all over her. Sometimes we'll wrestle a little, and push each other around. It never gets rough, although we've gotten accidental bumps and bruises. Then, later, she'll calm me down and I'll be softer."

A style is a particular way of doing things, and your sexual style is generally a reflection of the kind of person you are.

Shy: This person finds it hard to initiate sex, uses euphemisms instead of explicit language, and tends to follow what their partner wants. It's important for shy lovers to be sure they really want to do what their partner suggests.

Thoughtful: For thoughtful people, sex is much more than just a physical act, and so it must be prepared for, nurtured, and cultivated. These individuals often feel that the sexual act is a spiritual act and cannot be entered into lightly.

Gregarious: Sex may be part of something else, a need to communicate or an exuberant desire to express happiness. This type of person can lead or follow pretty easily.

Smoldering: When their sexual interest is sparked, they are consumed by it, and it's hard for them to think about anything else. They cannot divide their sexuality from the rest of life, and partners may find their style either appealing or overwhelming. A smoldering lover may lead or follow—sometimes it's the "come hither look" in the eye that makes the partner initiate sex.

Bossy: This person thinks about himself or herself first and may come on too brusquely to a partner. This style can be a real turn-on to some people, particularly shy individuals who have trouble expressing their sexual needs.

Most people tend to be a little of one, a little of another, mixed together in a unique hodge-podge. You may feel shy with some lovers but smoldering with others. Sometimes your mood or the day or the circumstance directs your actions and feelings.

Sex for One: How to Love Yourself

Portnoy had a right to complain! Why should people have been castigated throughout the centuries for making themselves feel good? And yet, the ancient Eastern religions as well as ancient Christian philosophers admonish us against "sinful, unnatural behavior." "Self-abuse," to me, implies some sort of terrible mutilation or punishment—yet this is exactly what our parents and grandparents called it.

Most of us have a lot of healing to do around the topic of masturbation. Why was giving yourself pleasure such a heinous crime? Because it meant you were wasting that precious stuff that could have been starting up a new generation. Because you were rebelling against those who would deem any kind of physical joy a crime, if it wasn't in the context of family, church, and state.

But let me come forward right now and proclaim the joys and benefits of masturbation:

- It feels good.

- It is the only assuredly safe form of physical (as opposed to mental) sex.

- It teaches you how your body works.

- It teaches you about pleasure.

- It shows you that you are an independent being.

- It is a testing ground for significant fantasies that may teach you a great deal about yourself and may serve to expand your imagination sexually and otherwise.

- It can be used as a form of meditation, bringing the body and mind into harmony together.

- For individuals who have no partner, it offers sexual release and all the benefits of pleasuring and orgasm described shortly.

- For individuals who have a partner, it offers a different sexual experience, one where you control everything and get exactly what you want each time.

In our teen years, there is nothing more exciting and sometimes frightening than our changing, volatile bodies, ready to explode at the slightest touch or pressure. One woman interviewed for the book said that when she was bored in junior high school, she would just cross her legs and squeeze her PC muscles and take herself to another realm. One woman who had been abused by her father told me that masturbation was her own form of comforting herself—for many years, she could have an orgasm by herself although she couldn't have one with a man.

Masturbation in adolescence repeats in a more sophisticated way the kind of physical exploration we did as toddlers. Of course, if our mother or father slapped that stroking hand away and yelled bloody murder when we were small, we may use masturbation in adolescence as a way to get back at our all-powerful parents.

Now, how do we get around the guilt trip over doing it? Let's examine this for a minute. People feel lousy about feeling good because they were told from a young age that you're not supposed to feel that good, ever. Physical pleasure was supposed to be evil or self-destructive (the madness-and-hairy-palms theory). And so, even as we discovered that we could feel free and joyous, we were thinking it wasn't so good to fly like this because we might get to enjoy it too much, and then what . . .?

Then real life would pale in comparison. Or maybe we'd spoil ourselves masturbating and not really like sex with a partner. If your strong right hand or your vibrator is the best lover you ever had, what do you need people for?

The answer, of course, is that people offer love and bonding and a relationship and all those good things. Masturbation is for pleasure, pure and simple. It's sex without love, orgasm without commitment or recrimination. But you must love yourself enough to enjoy this wonderful experience, and the more you experiment, the more you will reap the benefits of this solitary passion.

Men get to touch their genitals every time they urinate, and little boys even do it in groups. Contests for who can pee the farthest are common—after all, if you've got the equipment, you might as well use it. And masturbation is also a rite of passage for boys, who sometimes even gang up for jerk-off contests.

It is a much bigger deal for women. Not only do we gingerly wipe ourselves "in that area" (and many vaginal infections spring up because young girls are so busy trying not to make any physical contact with themselves, even with a toilet paper barrier in between), we have trouble touching the place or even talking about touching. To get to the pleasure part, we must explore an area that for many has been hidden and covered since we were in diapers.

Many women have no idea where their clitoris is or how it's shaped, or how much room there is between the urethral and vaginal openings or what lies in between the vagina and the anus. We never actually examine that district—which we could easily do by using a mirror when we masturbate. It's wonderful just to see the change in color in the labia, or the lubrication issuing from the vaginal opening.

Men will very often use a real physical image—a pornographic movie or magazine will nearly always bring a man to climax. For women, it is more commonly the pictures we paint in our brain that turn us on. This mental activity "incites us to sex," as Bill put it. The fantasies we conjure up during masturbation (see Chapter Ten for a full explanation of erotic daydreams) may make many of us cringe because of their violent or bizarre nature. A feminist may have a rape fantasy; a happily married newlywed may fantasize a ménage-à-trois; a woman may imagine herself with a penis; a man may see himself tied to the railroad tracks, being held down and subdued by another man and a dog.

It's all allowed. As a matter of fact, it's healthy to think these thoughts and enhance your masturbatory experiences. It means you are loving yourself well. Remember, having the fantasy doesn't mean you're perverted or are about to do devastating things to your neighbors. Fantasies live in the mind—most people do not change their behavior because of them.

Sensitivity Exercise for One

First Week: How do you allow yourself to fantasize and masturbate for a full, rich sexual experience? Give yourself plenty of time alone to explore your mind and body. Start with your clothes on, in a comfortable spot, and turn on some music. Allow your hands to roam freely over your body, experimenting with different forms of touch—light and teasing, insistent and repetitive, pushing, pulling, kneading, stroking, pinching. Avoid the genitals completely for now.

Direct your mind to the area of your body being touched and focus on the sensations you are having. See what thoughts and memories are triggered by that touch. Then let it go.

Move to a new area of your body. Let your mind travel with you, then expand it outward to a new visualization.

Be gentle; then rougher with yourself. See if your imagery changes when your touch changes.

If you are very aroused, let go of the physical contact and be very still, but see if you can continue the fantasy. When the feeling of imminent orgasm passes, resume the touch.

Practice this exercise daily *without bringing yourself to orgasm* for one week. At the end of the week, make a diary of the fantasies that you've had that seem most stimulating to you.

Second Week: Begin your sessions fully clothed. You may now include your genitals in the touch sequence. See if your fantasies escalate when you touch nipples, vulva, penis, testicles, anus.

As you become more excited, you may remove some of your clothing, but not all of it at once. See if you can include this disrobing in your visualization. What does it do to your sense of pleasure?

As you begin to approach orgasm, stop the touch. Take the time to remove all your clothing, slowly and sensuously, as though you were doing a striptease for a lover.

When you are naked, look at yourself in front of a full-length mirror and begin the touch sequence. Women will need a handheld mirror as well, to see what they really look like when they become aroused. What fantasies do you have, looking at yourself like this?

Begin the touch sequence again. Remember to include all your body areas now—not only the genitals. This way you can prolong the pleasure experience. Each time you approach orgasm, see if you can stop yourself. Contract your pubococcygeal muscles to stimulate and enhance the experience. The control you achieve over your own body while you are alone should give you a great sense of self-satisfaction, self-awareness, and power.

At last, allow yourself to come. (See below Questions and Answers About Orgasm.) If you continue the stimulation, even after your first peak, you may be able to generate several more. Even if you don't, keep up the touch. If you love yourself well, you need to stay with your feelings and fantasies even after the climax.

You may vary this sensitivity exercise in dozens of creative ways.

- *Position*: Masturbate standing, sitting, and lying down.

- *Temperature:* Experiment with the temperature of the room being warm or cool, while you are covered with a quilt or open to the air.

- *Use fabrics*: Experiment with the feel of different fabrics moving across your body.

- *Try a sex aid*: You may wish to use a vibrator or dildo, *ben wa* balls, or some other sex aid.

- After you've worked on the sensitivity exercises for a while, go back to your fantasy diary and see how it's expanded. You may find that you have become quite a poet, expressing your sexual desires, needs and enjoyment as you never have before—because you finally feel comfortable with it.

Enjoy yourself. This body is yours for a long, long time—treat it well.

Sex for Two:
How to Extend Your Sexual Health with a Partner

Here is the question of a lifetime: How do you make love to another person and have that experience heal your mind and body and enhance your good health?

Basically, what you do with someone else is a field trip into the unknown. You surrender control and at the same time, you take control. You follow and you lead. You concentrate and you forget everything you ever learned. That's good sex.

Why is it good for you? Aside from all the physical benefits mentioned elsewhere in this book, a sexual experience with another person is an opportunity to give all of yourself without putting up any fences or barriers. If you get good at it, you can be the ultimate altruist—constantly donating good feelings and good wishes to another *at the same time getting it all back for yourself.* If you are really into self-expression, the sexual act is the best time to speak your very own language of being. You are making another person feel good by what you do to them and also by how you appreciate their efforts to please you. If you can see just how much you've turned your lover on, you are enormously turned on yourself by seeing their excitement.

How do you become this all-giving, all-receiving leader/follower? You take the exercises described above and do them with your partner. Known in sexual therapy circles as *sensate focus* exercises, these planned times with a partner allow you to forget the goal of orgasm or the excitement of conquest and just feel good about feeling good.

Think about this: It is possible that, ever since you became a sexual being, you have been starting your sexual adventures from the end instead of the beginning.

Let us think of the way most teenagers go about their fumbling, furtive sex. They get in a car or go to some other semiprivate place, and they kiss a lot, they do some "necking" in the area of the neck and shoulders, then they work their way down the body in the activity known as "petting," and then, usually, they proceed directly to intercourse. Going right from kissing to penetration, especially for young women who are not prepared or lubricated or aroused, is going to be disappointing, difficult, and possibly painful. It will probably be disappointing for the young man, too, since, lacking experience in controlling his ejaculation, he'll have an urgent need to come immediately. The party will be over before it even begins.

So this A-to-Z sexual experience falls flat for both of them because jumping from the first step to the last without any of the intermediate steps defies the leisurely perusal of intimacy. But the more you practice sex this way, the more ingrained it becomes. And it's hard to change fixed habits.

If you have spent all your attention on your genitalia and your partner's, you are going about the process backward. In your sensate focus, at first, *you will avoid the genitals completely*. You need to become sensually aware with your partner to become sexually aware later on. This is the most beneficial healing process and will afford you a deeper understanding of your own and your lover's needs.

One woman interviewed for this book said that she felt the greatest secret of heterosexual lovemaking was lesbian sex, where there was no particular drive toward penetration. The whole body, mind, and spirit of each partner became a testing ground with which to invent and experiment. Sex toys , fingers, and tongues were used inside and outside the body, in no particular order.

In any sexual encounter where it's expected that one body part fit inside another (between a man and a woman or between two men), both partners tend to fall back into the old pattern of stepwise progression—from a little excitement and intimacy, to a little more and finally, at the top of the staircase, whammo, intercourse occurs to create the *big explosive sexy testosterone orgasm* (known in some circles as the B.E.S.T. orgasm).

But if heterosexuals and gay men could achieve the kind of circular, suspenseful, exploratory sex that two women have together, they would find that they could extend lovemaking longer and derive a lot more from it. You don't have to be a lesbian to discover the subtle permutations of all those steps in between A and Z. It's not what you do but who you are and what you feel.

This is certainly not to denigrate the role of the penis in lovemaking. The penis is a wonderful organ, the original shape-shifter, the tool of teasing and pulse of power. However, it is not the whole deal, or even half the deal. In our new orientation toward exploratory sex, the idea is not to focus entirely on putting a penis inside a vagina or an anus. There are many, many other things to do with it, and if you let your imagination fly, you will find them.

Sensitivity Exercise for Two

First week: Take half an hour with your partner where you can simply be together, clothed, touching, and fantasizing together (aloud if you choose). One partner remains completely passive; the other is the giver. As the giver, you may do or say anything to your partner as long as it isn't harmful or unpleasant. Do not touch the genitals at all. After fifteen minutes, switch places. If either of you feels that you are approaching orgasm, stop and let the feelings subside.

During the second half of the week, you may remove some of your clothing, but not all of it at once. See if you can include this disrobing in your visualization. What does it do to your sense of pleasure? To your partner's? Don't touch each other's genitals. You are finding out where your other erogenous zones are and how they react when touched in different ways.

I cannot say it too often: The most powerful sexual organ is the mind. The more you use your mind—the thinking part, the memory part, the visualization and imagery part, the communication part—the more thrilling your sex life will be.

Second week: Once again, alternate giving and receiving pleasure. You may now touch all parts of the body—as long as you don't concentrate on the genitals but give equal opportunities to every part of your lover, from skin to hair to the backs of knees. When you are receiving touch, keep your mind on that area and focus on the sensations you are having. See what thoughts and memories are triggered by that touch. Then let it go. Follow your partner's touch; let your mind go with it. Expand your fantasies and see if your imagery changes when your partner's touch changes from teasing to deliberate to fleeting to rough.

If you are very aroused, let go of the physical contact and be very still, but see if you can continue the fantasy. When the feeling of imminent orgasm passes, resume the touch.

Practice this exercise daily *without bringing your partner to orgasm* for one week. Each of you must tell the other if you're about to come so that you can let go of the touch. Women and gay men will probably have to use the stop-start technique for their male partners.

How to Delay the Male Orgasm with the Stop-Start Technique

When a man feels an orgasm coming, there is a point beyond which he can't stop it. Practice alone and with a partner will teach you where that point of inevitability is. Just before you've reached it, you must consciously relax your genital area. An orgasm can be triggered by a contraction of the buttocks or pelvis, so to prevent it, you have to ride the wave of your arousal but not allow it to take over. Counter the relaxed feeling in the lower half of your body by pressing the tip of your tongue against the roof of your mouth.

In order to delay your ejaculation with the stop-start technique, start by masturbating with a dry hand. When you feel you're about to come, stop the stimulation. Repeat this process until you're able to stave off ejaculation for fifteen minutes. When you can manage this, use a lubricant, which will enhance the sensitivity of your penis and make it harder for you to keep from coming. Once again, repeat the stop-start procedure until you're in control for fifteen minutes.

Next, let your partner help. First she will masturbate you with a dry, and then, with a lubricated hand, just as you've done yourself. Finally, you can try this inside your partner. It's best to have her on top, so that you can guide her hips with your hands and tell her when to stop moving. When the urge to come has passed, she can start being active again. When you can go for fifteen minutes inside her, allow yourself to come.

How to Delay the Female Orgasm

This is usually not a big problem—most women spend most of their lives trying to figure out how to come, not how to prevent coming. However, for the purposes of this exercise, you want to bring yourself to the point of orgasm and then stop stimulation. In this way, you can ride the waves of pleasure even longer.

Relax your body completely. Your partner may stimulate your breasts and nipples or your vulva until you are sufficiently hot and bothered. Now contract your PC muscles, take a big breath, and imagine the arousal racing from the center of your body, to your genitals then to your anus and up your spinal column to the top of your head. You may feel a wonderful current coursing through you that feels similar to but less pressured and demanding than an orgasm.

Third week: Before you begin your lovemaking sessions, turn each other on by talking about the fantasies that you've had that are most stimulating to you. Refer to the fantasy diary you've been keeping for masturbation for inspiration. As you make contact with each other, see if your fantasies escalate when you touch nipples, vulva, penis, testicles, anus.

Take the time to remove each other's clothing, examining the sheen of the body as it comes into view. Enjoy the partially clothed body; then enjoy the naked body with its lovely display of skin running from top to toes. How does it feel along your fingertips? Does your partner get goosebumps when you touch certain areas?

When you are naked, look at yourselves without touching, using only your eyes to become aroused. What fantasies do you have, looking at your partner like this? Being looked at like this?

Begin the touch sequence again. Remember to include all your body areas now—not only the genitals. This way you can prolong the pleasure experience. You may wish to bring your partner to orgasm or to come yourself, or you may wish to delay it. Don't plan—do what comes naturally.

When you do come, continue the stimulation, even after your first peak. You may be able to generate several orgasms, and even if you don't, the prolonged contact with your partner offers you more benefit in terms of its calming, soothing effect. The sexual act is not completed until the body relaxes and returns to its unaroused state. If you care about yourself and your partner, you need to stay with your feelings and fantasies even after the climax.

Do experiment with positions—standing, sitting, and lying. Experiment with the feel of different fabrics moving across your body, with the temperature of the room being warm or cool, while you are covered with a quilt or open to the air. You may wish to use a vibrator or dildo, or some other sex aid.

Including Sex Toys and Useful Foods in Your Love Play

Dildos and vibrators used to be unmentionables relegated to XXX-rated movies. But, today, sex toys are increasingly popular aids to expand your sexual horizons, and are available in some drug-stores and sex shops, through mail-order catalogs, and through home parties, similar to those given to sell plastic food containers. The reason for this proliferation of sexual paraphernalia is simple: new relationships *require* safer sex practices, and many of these items offer either protection against disease transmission or provide a novel way to have fun without putting you or your partner at risk.

If you are in a committed, mutually monogamous relationship, you may wish to stimulate new areas of exploration with a partner. You can find an assortment of goodies to help you out:

- Condoms in every color, flavor and texture, for males.
- The Reality condom for females (see Chapter Five). There must be some creative couples who will get into the erotic natrue of this device.
- Dental dams, 6-inch-square pieces of latex for oral sex.
- Erotic underwear including edible panties.
- Creams and water-based lotions for massage and lubrication.
- Dildos for the vagina and anus, in different lengths and thick-nesses.
- Vibrators, also of accommodating sizes, with different speeds. Some have attachments so that you can insert them in two ori-fices at once.
- Specially strung beads for inserting, then pulling slowly out of orifices.
- Movies to watch at home to inspire you and set you afire (most of these are rather dull after the first viewing!)

See the Resource Guide for addresses of mail-order catalogs where you can purchase these items.

Food is an often overlooked but excellent sensual appetizer to a healthy sex life (although some of the best foods for sex are high in calories and fat!) You'll need to put a towel underneath you and will probably want to take a shower or bath afterward, but that's another lovely sensual thing to do together.

Here's what you may want to have in stock:

For a mutually monogamous couple who don't need a condom:

- Whipped cream
- Peanut butter (smooth variety)
- Ice cream
- Chocolate sauce
- Nonfat yogurt
- Maple (and other) syrup
- Honey or jam
- Ricotta cheese
- Bananas
- Liqueurs

For a nonmutually monogamous couple, only water-based items are allowed. Oil-based foods and animal fats can tear the latex in a condom or dam. Your list includes:

- Honey
- Jellies
- Syrups
- Powdered sugar
- Ice cubes/hot packs depending on weather
- Wine or champagne

This food and drink can be smeared on all parts of the body and licked off. You can put some in your mouth and feed some to your partner in a kiss. One clever couple favor cannolis, those wonderful Italian tube-shaped pastries filled with vanilla cream. She feeds him the cream, then fits the cannoli shell on his penis and eats it off him. (These shells are typically narrower than most erect penises and must be stretched a little to fit.)

Anything and everything belongs in a good sexual encounter. Remember, you are satisfying an appetite of one sort when you make love, and combining this with other appetites—for food, music, fine art (fingerpainting on your partner is cool), warmth, cold, light, dark—it all fits perfectly.

Lubrication:
The Way to Keep
Sexually Active at Any Age

When we're very young, we have all the lubrication we need—our joints are flexible, our mouths water, and we create natural secretions during the sexual act that allow us to remain comfortable even with a lot of friction and rubbing. As we get older, however—for some, this may occur in the thirties, some in the forties, and some in the fifties—we start drying up. This is true of both men and women, however, sexually, it affects women more specifically. Our hormonal time clock has a lot to do with vaginal dryness. And other factors, such as nervousness and fear, may also make it impossible for us to lubricate.

Couples tend not to discuss this, but invasive sex can be very painful for both parties if the woman isn't wet enough. One excellent way to stave off dryness is to use saliva as a lubricant, whether or not you're having oral sex. Another great idea is to do things that are noninvasive. If you aren't sticking one body part inside another, you don't have to worry as much about lubrication.

However, if you are having vaginal or certainly anal sex with a partner, you need to grease up:

- KY Jelly is an old standard, perfectly useful though it may make you think of your doctor's office.

- Replens is an over-the-counter preparation that comes in applicator form—the woman injects herself with a dollop of this before sex. Other OTC brands are GyneMoistrin, Lubrin, and Today Personal Lubricant.

- Astroglide is an excellent slippery lubricant that feels just like the body's natural secretions. It comes in tubes and bottles and is available in many sex shops.

- Egg white is a great natural product to use during sex to get you wetter.

- Unflavored unpasteurized yogurt protects you from yeast infections and lubricates as well—but is not water-based, and therefore is perilous to the safety of a condom.

You Don't Have to Be Past Fifty to Need a Lubricant

Many people think they don't have to be concerned about lubrication until after their fiftieth birthday. Not true! Young people tend to be very tight and anxious prior to sex, and lubrication can actually change the mood. Applying a substance to your partner or watching them apply it to themselves can also be a turn-on. Jack, our concert pianist who didn't masturbate until he was in his twenties, couldn't bring himself to orgasm until his roommate suggested using a lubricant. From the first try, it was a success.

Use Time, Place, and Mood for Greater Sexual Pleasure

You can have great sex anywhere. It can be fast or slow, a quickie or a day in bed. It's always most pleasurable if you coordinate what you want with your partner.

Indoors

Explore different rooms. What would you do in the bath together? In the kitchen on the table, maybe on pillows in a windowseat. What could you use to elevate the sensory awareness of your experience? Candles, music or tapes of natural sounds, incense, and different fabrics are all mood-enhancers.

Outdoors

Make sure you're comfortable. You want to take advantage of the fresh air, the soft grass, a flat rock, a sheltering tree, the sounds of crickets and birds, the dappled sunlight, or soft rain. Comment on it; make use of it.

Moving your sex life into a sensual life will expand your feelings about one another into the world around you. When you are not just a couple, but part of a larger whole, you have the potential to experience sex as a deeper, more spiritual event. When you are fused with everything around you, you may start to feel that your sex life is a lot more than just a collection of body parts colliding in space.

A Prescription for Good Sex for Two

The suggestions that follow can serve as springboards for your own creativity. You can use my ideas and enhance them as you become more expert and daring with your sexuality. Take one or two of these at a time, or the whole list, day or night, whenever the mood strikes. Play together; rest together; treat each other well.

- Start with an erotic massage session, completely clothed.
- Undress each other, stopping to revel in each body part you expose.
- Skip the candlelit dinner and instead opt for foods of great texture and taste (avocado, peanut butter, or whipped cream) eaten off your partner's body.
- Now you're sticky. Go give each other a bath and hairwash.
- Pile towels on the floor and dry each other by rolling around together in the towels (it doesn't matter that you just got so clean).
- Peel off the towels and get into bed or onto a couch. See how many parts of your lover's body you can kiss without going near the genitals. Spend a long time on earlobes, toes, elbows, knees.
- Never go for the gold. When you see that you are driving your partner wild, extend the experience by leaving whatever you are doing temporarily and going on to something else. Then come back to whatever it was that really excited your partner and see if you can bump that ecstasy up another notch.
- Sometimes, keep yourself from coming. Stay with the moment, squeeze your PC muscles, inhale deeply and hold the breath, change position, concentrate on your partner. See if you can get

a wave of pleasure instead of a bona fide orgasm. Next time, you can come.

- If you aren't having orgasms and want to have them, stick with one motion, slow and repetitive, for a period of time. Women, don't worry about taking too long—your partner won't get bored. If it takes an hour, so be it. But if your partner is giving you a type of stimulation that isn't stimulating, say something (nicely, see Chapter Six). Men, you may have to guide your partner as to how you like your penis stimulated, particularly if you want oral or manual stimulation. It won't hurt your partner's feelings if you explain how to use rhythmic stroking with both hands or with the mouth and hands (put your partner's finger in your mouth to demonstrate if you need to).

- If you decide to have intercourse, don't make it the last thing you do. Go on and use your mouths or other orifices. Use everything you've got.

- Talk, laugh, play, press each other's buttons.

How to Keep Sexuality at Its Peak After Making Love

Here you are in the bedroom. You have been rolling around together for a couple of hours; you have both come (perhaps several times) and you are basically exhausted. Maybe you doze a little. But you are awake, and filled with yourself and your lover. Maybe you feel like your insides have been warmed by firelight and you are suffused with peace.

Think of the sexual act as just a piece of what the two of you are doing now, lying together, and what you may do tomorrow or did the day before yesterday. Your sexuality is like the roots of a tree, spreading as deeply underground as the branches extend on top.

The afterglow and closeness between you—even if you are not life-mates, is exceptionally important to your sexual health. It is only when we feel continuity in life that we are able to consolidate body, mind and spirit. Sometimes, you may just wish to lie silent, thinking your own thoughts, staring off into space.

But this is a terrific opportunity to talk about things you rarely discuss. Several people interviewed for this book said that after the sexual act was over, they often talked about their childhood, their work or lack of it, their aspirations for the future, their fears about the imminent death of a parent. Coming together with a partner has given you a brief glimpse into how good things can get. Why not bring that awareness into a bigger arena? If you trust your partner to open every orifice of your body and give it delight, why not trust that person one step further?

Make a deal to rebound off your physical relationship into another important set of agendas. Talk it out.

- Maybe you have a problem with a friend or relative you've kept quiet about for a long time that your partner could offer suggestions about.

- Maybe your partner has been feeling self-conscious because of a weight problem or some chronic ailment and you could assuage some of the difficult feelings.

- Maybe the two of you have been thinking about selling the house, or changing jobs or making a radical financial move—yet you haven't shared the particulars. This is the time to do it.

Sex is a creative venture, but it can grow even more healthful and life-sustaining after you stop making love.

Questions and Answers *About Orgasm*

It has been described, poetically, as flying. As spontaneous eruption, like a volcano. As if you've burst out of your skin and are only partly back inside it. As if you're inside a raging fire, carried on the pounding waves of the ocean, catapulting into outer space. But what is it, really?

Q: What is an orgasm?

A: An orgasm is the body's mechanism for the release of physical tension that mounts up due to sexual stimulation and the excitement that this titillating experience causes. Orgasms are unique to individuals—for some, they are gentle waves of pleasure, for others, cataclysmic vibrations that shake the mind and body.

Prior to orgasm, of course, must come desire. If we had no inclination toward sexual release, our bodies would not begin to react. Desire may come from fantasy (imagined scenarios or wished sexual encounters), from sensory stimulation (seeing a picture of a partly clothed body, smelling a perfume, brushing past someone on the subway), or from an actual erotic suggestion made by another person.

Once desire has taken hold of us, we are mesmerized by sex. We think about it frequently, often in conjunction with other thoughts, we are distracted from less exciting activities, we feel a heaviness and wetness in the genitals if we're female and a tingling in the testicles or a partial erection if we're males.

If we desire sex, we can act on it or not. If we do act, there are the famous four steps toward release, described by Masters and Johnson in their landmark work, *Human Sexual Response*.

1. *Excitement phase*. During this phase, a variety of physical changes take place, both in the genitals and the body as a whole. In both men and women, there is generally a flush or reddening in the upper body, an experience of voluntary muscle tension in the genitals and anus, and very often, blood pressure, heartbeat, perspiration, and respiration increase.

2. *Plateau phase*. This stage takes all the earlier reactions to a higher level, and in addition, definite genital changes occur. The penis increases in circumference and its color deepens. All men gain about three inches in length when they reach a full erection—the smaller the flaccid penis, the greater the proportion of growth. The testes enlarge to a 50 percent increase over their unstimulated state, and the nipples are often erect as well. A shut-off mechanism prevents the escape of urine through the ureter.

For women, the clitoris comes front and center, emerging from its hiding place under the hood, the uterus rises and vagina becomes wider and deeper, forming a tent or depression where the semen can collect. There's a great deal of lubrication along the rugal folds (the accordionlike ridges of the vaginal barrel). The labia are engorged with venous blood and there is a vivid color change ranging from bright red to deep wine for women who have borne children and from light to deep pink in childless women. The nipples become erect if they have not done so already.

3. *Orgasm.* The culmination of the two prior phases is orgasm, that feeling of being swept away. Some people feel they are about to faint as they are overcome by waves of pleasure. For a woman, there are four origins of orgasm:

- Orgasm in the clitoral area
- Orgasm in the vaginal/uterine area (usually from stimulation of the Grafenberg or G-spot which can be felt through the front vaginal wall)
- Orgasm stemming from a blend of the two
- Orgasm generated by fantasy and visualization only, with no stimulation of the body

Most reports indicate that the clitoral-centered orgasm is a faster, more immediately exhilarating experience than the slow, delicious buildup to the vaginal–uterine orgasm. The blended orgasm and "mind" orgasm have elements of both of the other types.

During the female orgasm, the vagina and uterus experience contractions that vary in intensity. Some women may experience a small, brief peak with an immediate return to plateau; some may have sequential orgasms, different peaks separated by short breaks; still others may have multiple orgasms, as one after another peak is reached without ceasing.

For a man, the pleasure of orgasm is twofold.

After a sufficient amount of stimulation, the autonomic nervous system begins to secrete adrenalin or norepinephrine from the brain down the spinal column, dividing in half around the back muscles and, finally, to the genitals. The penis and testicles, as well as the glands and muscles surrounding these organs, are washed in neurotransmitter stimulation.

a. *emission phase:* The set of signals from the nerves squeezes the muscles that send the sperm to the prostate. In this phase, the prostate and surrounding muscles contract, the testes move close to the body and pressure in the seminal fluid rises. The man knows at this point that ejaculation is inevitable.

   b. *propulsion phase:* During the second stage, the nerves order another set of muscle contractions. The penis itself begins to contract rhythmically when the outer urethral sphincter opens and seminal fluid (semen and sperm) rushes out.

   During climax, the anal sphincter contracts, the whole body may go rigid, and the thumbs and big toes straighten while fingers and other toes bend upward.

4. *Resolution.* The body slowly regains its predesire lack of tension and anticipation. We feel satiated, comfortable, at ease in our partner's arms. Sometimes, we're so relaxed, we fall asleep.

Q: How much semen do you lose in a normal ejaculation?

A: About a teaspoon's worth; however this amount can multiply by four if you haven't had a sexual encounter in a long time.

Q: Do orgasms occur naturally or are they learned experiences?

A: They don't occur naturally to all women, and there may also be men who have to "practice" their orgasmic capacity. Through a variety of techniques, first in masturbation, then with a partner, you can teach yourself to have an orgasm (or have more orgasms if you are already orgasmic). By doing graded stimulation exercises, using your hand or a vibrator, you can bring yourself almost but not quite to peak. When the sensations begin to subside, you can stimulate yourself again to the brink of pleasure—or allow yourself full release. In this way, you can teach yourself how to be orgasmic.

Q: Is there a difference between orgasms from masturbation and orgasms from coitus?

A: There are all kinds of orgasms, some that are like a sighing breath and some that are like a raging bull. There are those you barely perceive and those that apparently go on for a quarter of an hour. However, clinically, an orgasm is an orgasm is an orgasm—there is no difference in physiological response. A clitorally-based orgasm is no less "good" or "legitimate" than a vaginal–uterine–based orgasm. An orgasm a man gives himself with a hand job can be as pleasurable as one from a partner's blow job or from ejaculating inside his partner. Each orgasm depends on the situation, the timing, and the frame of mind in which it takes place.

Many individuals interviewed said that they experience a more intense, deeper, and sometimes more unself-conscious orgasm when they're alone and don't have to worry about pleasing a partner. Women do report a difference in sensation, depending on where their orgasm is based (see the earlier discussion) and both men and women talk about some orgasms that bond them so securely to the person they love, it feels as though they have experienced their partner's orgasms as well as their own.

Q: Does the cervix "feel" the penis hitting against it?

A: The tip of the cervix is abundant with nerve endings, so for many women, the feeling of contact with the penis causes enormous pleasure. Animal studies have shown that nerve impulse stimuli generated from penile thrusting against the cervix can trigger the release of FSH and LH, the pituitary hormones that regulate the female menstrual cycle. A woman who has had a hysterectomy where the cervix must be removed along with the uterus must adjust to the loss of this experience during sex. A sexually active woman who is undergoing this operation should always inform her surgeon that she wants the vaginal cuff sewn down as far as possible, offering as much room in the vagina as can be afforded. Men who have a small penis may be self-conscious about "filling the space"; however, since the vagina is a completely elastic organ, it changes shape to fit whatever's inside it. (You can test this yourself by putting one finger only about three or four inches up the vagina and touching the cervix.)

Q: Do you always know when you're having an orgasm?

A: Men nearly always know, even if they don't ejaculate when they come. (This is true of young boys who have dry orgasms, elderly men whose ejaculate is very scanty, and any age man who is on medication or has a chronic condition that would affect the ejaculate).

Many women claim they've never had an orgasm because they don't know what they're "supposed" to feel. You can probably say you've had one with some assurance if, during the sexual act, you experience a buildup of tension, a peak, and then a gradual return to a relaxed state. A person who's been brought up to believe that sex is dirty or that she isn't worthy to receive so much pleasure may stop herself from getting to the orgasmic stage. A tender partner or a good therapist might be able to convince her to surrender and let go of her emotions.

Some men talk about orgasm as an explosion, either inside or outside. Some women describe having an orgasm as "being turned inside out." Others talk about having shivers, their breath stopping, their heart pounding, their voice rising to a banshee scream. Some say that they can feel their womb shift during the moment of release, and in fact, there is a mechanism that raises the uterus during arousal. Anything and everything is possible, permissible, and usually wonderful.

There are, however, women who experience pain during intercourse and men who are unable to have an erection sufficient for orgasmic release—this may be physiological or psychological or a combination of both (see Chapter Nine for possible causes)—but a sensitive physician or therapist can help with this problem.

Q: *What's the G-spot and how do I stimulate it?*

A: The Grafenberg spot (G-spot), named by sex researchers John Perry, Ph.D. and Beverly Whipple, Ph.D., R.N. for Dr. Ernst Grafenberg, the physician who located it in 1950, is a sensitive area that can be felt through the front wall of the vagina between the pubic bone and the opening to the vaginal canal. You can locate this spot—if you have long fingers—by reaching beyond the pubic bone and pressing upward. As you stimulate it, you will notice that it swells—in some women, to the size of a half–dollar. It's been described as a "small spongy bean." It may be easier for a partner to identify the spot manually first, so that you can both determine where it is. Your partner can reach it best during intercourse or manual stimulation from a rear-entry position.

If you wish to find it for yourself, try sitting on the toilet after urinating and reach up along the front wall, pushing up toward your belly button. Take your other hand and press down on your abdomen just above the pubic bone. At first it may feel as though you have to urinate again, but if you allow the feeling to increase, you will find that you can experience a great deal of sexual pleasure.

Stimulation of the G-spot typically makes a woman first feel as though she is going to urinate, and she may in fact ejaculate a fluid that looks like skim milk mixed with water. The pleasurable sensations caused by pressure on this spot travel along the pudendal nerve and sacral plexus to the spinal cord.

Q: *Can men experience multiple orgasms?*

A: Yes, although few do. Kinsey found that only 15 to 20 percent of men in their teens and twenties had multiple orgasms. A more recent study shows that the group who enjoyed the most multiple climaxes were in their forties, and a third were fifty-five or older. In other words, sex *can* get better as you get older and more experienced. It may take years for a man to gain control over his ejaculations.

To inhibit ejaculation (which would end the orgasmic experience), multiorgasmic men contract their PC muscles (pubococcgeal muscles, between the testes and the anus), and use breathing and different postures to "hold" the experience and allow it to occur again. Some leakage of semen may occur during each orgasm, but if the man or his partner can continue stimulation while preventing himself from letting go, he can reach one peak after another, similar to what occurs in many women. If his prostate is stimulated (either by insertion of a lubricated finger in the anus or by applying pressure to the perineum), his orgasmic sensation may be heightened.

Q: *Do men and women need manual, oral, coital, or anal stimulation (i.e., some form of touch) to experience orgasm?*

A: Many women can give themselves an orgasm without touching any part of their body at all through visualization and fantasy.

A woman who has awakened from dreaming, aware that she has come in her sleep, is probably capable of the "thought orgasm." Although some women report they've always been able to bring themselves to a peak without any touch, this, too, can be a learned experience. It can be enhanced by performing Kegels (see Chapter Eight), which impart both health and pleasure benefits.

Almost all men experience nocturnal emissions, or wet dreams, as they pass through puberty, and it's also possible for a man to have an orgasm during the REM sleep cycle if he has an erotic dream. When awake, however, it's more than likely a man will touch himself or ask a partner to touch him if he wants to come.

Q: Why are erections good for you?

A: When the penis is flaccid, it receives less oxygen than any other body organ. But when erect, the muscle and nerve cells are nourished by the abundance of oxygenated blood pumping through its veins and arteries. Muscle cells stay far more elastic and supple when they get oxygen—which means that each erection guarantees that the next will be even firmer.

Q: Why is orgasm healthful?

A: There are so many reasons why orgasm is good for you! First, we all need to release our sexual tension. Not doing so, according to some experts, can cause headaches, joint pain, crankiness, exhaustion, and frustration. But there are a variety of other reasons:

- *During the process of excitement building to orgasm, the body lubricates itself.* When aroused, the Bartholin's glands in women and Cowper's glands in men begin to produce hormonal secretions. This is particularly beneficial after midlife, when estrogen and testosterone levels decline naturally. Since excitement and orgasm keep the female internal organs lubricated, the more the better.

- *Orgasm can allieviate pain.* In a 1985 study at Rutgers University conducted by Beverly Whipple, Ph.D., R.N., and Barry R. Komisaruk, Ph.D., volunteers were asked to stimulate themselves with a specially designed pressure transducer in a laboratory setting while undergoing painful finger compression. (This was done with a special device that squeezed a finger until the participant said, "pain.") The women in the study were able to tolerate significantly more pain when they pleasured themselves and even more when they achieved orgasm, than when they were simply distracted by other stimuli. A follow-up study in 1988 confirmed the fact that genital stimulation served as an analgesic against pain.

One reason for the pain-relief effect is that during orgasm, the brain produces endorphins, powerful natural painkillers similar to morphine in chemical structure. Other neurotransmitters mediate this effect, however, so this is not the whole explanation. Some of it has to do with redirected blood flow, away from the affected area to the genitals; a lot of it has to do with the brain and nervous system activity during sexual response. And some of it is emotionally based, as well.

Many individuals with crippling arthritis, whiplash and other painful conditions often find that they can enjoy hours of pain relief following orgasm (see Chapter Nine).

- *Orgasm enhances or restores your sense of well-being.* The release of tension after orgasm makes us tingle with pleasurable memories and physical comfort. This is often called "the glow," partly because of the flush caused by dilated blood vessels that lasts even after the sexual act is over. Being cherished and wanted makes us feel good about ourselves and the one we're with.

- *Orgasm has an indirect healing effect on a variety of conditions.* When you are distracted, you are less likely to concentrate on what ails you. The powerful stimulation of orgasm can at least temporarily alleviate stiffness, tension, headache and backache, and insomnia, and it may also positively affect such emotional problems as depression and anxiety.

- *Orgasm establishes closeness between partners.* Regardless of what's going on in your relationship, it is the odd couple who doesn't feel a certain bond after sharing this experience—it's kind of like a private joke that no one else in the room understands. When you have given to and received from someone else, you are solidifying a social interaction that may lead to other forms of intimacy. And you can be more intimate with each other in nonsexual ways after sharing an orgasm.

Q: *Where do most people feel their orgasms?*

A: When we first start having orgasms, they are pretty directly felt in the genitals—the penis for a man with possibly some tingling in the testes as well, the clitoris for a woman with some awareness of uterine or vaginal spasms as well.

As we grow more experienced sexually, we are likely to feel orgasm in a more global way. Women in particular report feeling that they come all over—from their nipples to their thighs, from the top of the head to their fingertips. This type of "holistic" orgasm is possible for men, too, but it very much depends on how attentive the couple is to stimulating and pleasuring nongenital areas of the body. One woman interviewed reported her first type of overall orgasm when her lover sucked on her toes and licked in between them.

Q: *What's the difference between a male and female orgasm?*

A: Winnifred Cutler, Ph.D., author of *Love Cycles* aptly describes it as the difference between a sneeze and a yawn. A sneeze is uncontrollable, it is expulsive, it races through the body but exits at one point. A yawn, on the other hand, tends to spread slowly and affect several organs—the mouth widens, the eyes tear, the respiration adjusts to a heaving sigh. The biggest difference, however, is that you can stifle a yawn. Many women have done this successfully for decades with their orgasms. This is one reason for the breach between one sex and the other—males commonly wanting to leap ahead toward climax, females needing a sufficient "warm-up" time during excitement and plateau for lubrication and other vaginal changes, and for feeling completely in the moment.

Q: *What prevents you from having orgasms?*

A: There are so many barriers that can hold us back from really enjoying ourselves sexually. Childhood or adolescent sexual trauma, old guilts, fear of discovery, false expectations, over-concern about our partner, distractions (from street noise to thinking about the bills), inappropriate touch, inability to ask for the kind of touch you want, a sense of being clumsy or ugly or awkward, and the biggest one of all—trying too hard! These and many more can stop us from having orgasms.

Q: *What if you're with an ungiving partner who can't bring you to orgasm?*

A: Nobody takes you anywhere you don't want to go. If you're not having orgasms, it's because you're inhibiting them at some level. Even when you have a wonderful lover who devotes enormous amounts of time and energy to helping you come, it is you who are in charge. You turn yourself on, even to the extent of being attracted to another individual. And you provide the orgasm (which you can prove to yourself by masturbating).

Q: *Why would we cry or laugh after having an orgasm?*

A: The release of physical and emotional tension may be so great as to cause a mixture of joy and pain—joy at having the experience of orgasm and sharing with another; pain of knowing that once this amazing bonding experience has ended, we are back to ground zero, separate individuals. And, too, there is an awareness after experiencing what the French call, *le petit mort* (the little death) that we are vulnerable to death itself. Occasionally, frustration about a not particularly satisfying sexual or emotional experience may make us laugh as a defensive tactic.

Q: *Is a simultaneous orgasm (both partners coming at the same time) an indication of a really good sexual relationship?*

A: Maybe yes, maybe no. People who are technical masters at controlling orgasms can simply time their climaxes together—this does give a great sense of fulfillment, but it may not mean very much emotionally. You may be too distracted, when pleasuring your partner, to take pleasure for yourself. For both people not to miss their moment, sometimes it's preferable to let one person come first, then the other.

Naturally, when both partners are involved simultaneously in giving and taking pleasure, the very excitement generated between you may cause you to come simultaneously—and this can be a rich, spiritual, meaningful love experience. But it's unwise to expect this to happen all the time—actually, simultaneous orgasms in couples are pretty rare.

Q: *I've heard that some people come in colors. Why does this happen and can you learn to do it?*

A: The brain chemistry is exceptionally sensitive during orgasm, and the stimulation of various neurotransmitters may affect the occipital lobe, which is responsible for vision. A sensitive individual may see a display that looks like a rainbow or fireworks; some report seeing other pictures during orgasm which may actually be visual memories. (We may say that people who have religious experiences, such as the whirling dervishes, or pilgrims, who see portentous omens at a shrine, are going through a similar mental process.) Other lobes of the brain may also be affected during orgasm—some people may hear music or feel the action of waves pulsing over their body.

You probably can't learn to do this; and if you're coming in colors now, you may not be forever. It's wonderful, of course, but best to take each experience as it happens and not try for it, or anticipate it. If you look forward to an orgasm so that you can have a particular vision, and it doesn't occur, you may be disappointed in the entire experience.

Q: *What are common fears about having an orgasm?*
- That you'll faint
- That you'll make unpleasant noises or faces
- That you will lose control, both physical and emotional (Many people fear they will become "slaves" to the one who helps them to have an orgasm.)
- That it will mean you're not a "good girl"
- That it will mean a woman is in charge of you—that you are "pussy-whipped" if you come when *she* wants you to
- That if you come too soon, she won't be satisfied.

Q: *Can men have an orgasm without an erection? Without ejaculation? Without the testes rising?*

A: Yes, to all three. A completely impotent man (that is, a man who never has an erection when aroused, or cannot sustain an erection long enough for penetration) can still experience the peak of orgasmic pleasure when he is stimulated either manually or orally. He may or may not ejaculate without an erection.

A man with an erection may have an orgasm without ejaculation, particularly if he controls the experience (see the discussion for multiorgasmic men).

Part of the normal physiological mechanism for male orgasm involves the involuntary response of the testes, which rise to sit close to the body. However, men with spinal cord injury who do not experience this effect can still have the feeling of an orgasm.

Q: *Does it take body knowledge to be really orgasmic?*

A: Since anything can stop an orgasm before it gets going, the more aware you are of your own body's responses, the easier it will be for you to have orgasms. Older women tend to be more orgasmic than younger women, and older men are more capable of having multiple orgasms than younger men. A valid reason is that they have more practice from having done this activity for a longer time.

Q: *If I've been faking orgasms, how can I stop doing that and still make my partner happy?*

A: Faking an orgasm is similar to telling people you own a palazzo on the Italian Riviera—you know it's a lie, they know it's a lie, and the entire ruse is futile. You do not make your partner happy by trying to "get away" with lying. The best course of action is to talk about the fact that whatever you're doing together does not arouse you sufficiently to come. Your partner will be much happier figuring out with you what you really want out of your sexual relationship.

Q: *Can you really enjoy sex if you're nonorgasmic?*

A: Certainly. Touch is a basic human need, and holding onto a partner, cuddling, stroking, kissing, and any other form of contact is beneficial. For people who have been abused in childhood or early adulthood, it may feel too overwhelming to let go in orgasm. Psychotherapy may be a passageway to overcoming blocks that stop us from being orgasmic; however, if we are comfortable enough with another person to allow touch, we are certainly on the right track.

Talking to Your Kids About Sex:

Building a Healthy Foundation

*W*e are light-years beyond the birds and bees, winging away on sophisticated concepts such as family life education, role modeling, and appropriate gender identification. And yet, down deep where it counts, we are still scared silly to talk about sex—or sexuality, which is harder—to our children. We are stuck in the same old, same old as our parents, hoping that the idea of sex will somehow find its way into our children's minds and hearts without our having to do anything. The most liberal-minded parents, with sometimes really excellent sex lives, pale at the notion of hearing their child ask, "Mommy, Daddy, why does it feel so good when I touch myself down here?"

Why can't we help them, whether our kids are toddlers or teens? The reason, of course, is that we have no models to work with. If our parents shut the door on us when they were naked, if they refused to name *all* our body parts, or gave us euphemisms for our genitalia, if they brandished the sword of hairy palms and mental derangement when we wanted to explore our "private parts," if they spewed out the messages that we could "get in trouble" from "having sex" when we were teens, well, no wonder we don't know how to tell our kids any better.

We know—and this is the really frightening part—that we have no control over those young, impressionable, curious minds. If we open the door just a little for them, anything and everything, from orgasm to homosexuality to condom usage, might go pouring in. And *then* what would we say, when they asked us if it was okay to experiment?

*G*et Clear About the Message Before You Send It

Regardless of your feelings, values, religious beliefs, and so on, here are the basics of what you need to convey to your child:

248

- We are all sexual from the beginning of our lives, at least from the first birthday.

- Sex is not an act but a way of being; it's part of our personality.

- There are stages of sexual intimacy—you can be incredibly close to someone without touching; then you can keep your space but enter another's if they say it's okay; and finally, you can combine physical attraction and genuine caring for each other by expressing yourself sexually.

Sex hygiene, like tooth-brushing and helmets for bike-riding, is a preventive health-care tactic. It must be reinforced time and again. I'm not trying to reduce joy and ecstasy to the banal acts that keep us safe from dental caries and broken heads, but I do want to stress that it's essential for kids to know that you have to mix in a big dollop of common sense with emotion and passion. This message has to come early on.

Daily exposure to matters sexual makes them less scary and intimidating. No, you shouldn't allow your child into your conjugal bed; you can, however, point out the copulating animals at the zoo and lead right into a discussion of fertility, contraception, and birth. Suppose you're watching TV together and there's an incident about a boy touching a girl's breasts. You can ask your child what he or she thinks about the situation, and even take it further, asking what he or she would do if they were one of the characters. Use situations from real life, books, the newspapers, anything that seems overtly or covertly sexual.

My eight-year-old daughter and I had a fascinating evening taking apart an old Dean Martin/Jerry Lewis film where Martin, trying to "get the girl," shoves her down on a sandy beach and forces himself on her in the tradition of good old, aggressive, masculine flirting. Martin's obnoxious physicality arose from the mind-set of, "This is what she really wants, but is just too timid to ask for."

As we watched, I grew angrier and complained about what a terrible, violent scene this was.

My perceptive child said, "It looks like he's hurting her, not kissing her, Mommy."

And this interchange allowed her to question the idea that a kiss wasn't always warm and mushy and nice. She ended by saying staunchly, with my approval, that she would never let anyone push her down and treat her like that.

You can play "what if" games with your kids to teach them refusal skills. You can model healthy affection by kissing your partner at any and every opportunity. And you can hug your kids all you like, which will communicate to them more than anything the delight and importance of touch.

Get Comfortable with Your Own Sexuality

If you cannot talk the talk, you cannot walk the walk. There is a reluctance in our society to say things to one another that are embarrassing, silly, or potentially humiliating, but that's exactly what we have to do when it comes to the subject of sexuality and kids.

If your child wants to know where she comes from, and your response is Cincinnati, or "the stork brought you," stop and think about your flip reply. It will turn the conversation off immediately, without quenching your child's thirst for the answer. She will know you're lying and go elsewhere, to her other parent, grandparent or close adult friend, or to another child, who may be less informed about sex than she is. So the cop-out only makes her feel, "my parents don't take me seriously. They won't talk about real things that concern me deeply."

Think for a minute about your own childhood. So many of us came from families where we didn't even see our parents hug or kiss, where girls thought they had a dread disease and were about to die as soon as they had their first period, where boys thought themselves bed-wetters after their first nocturnal emission. And there was *no one* to ask—you might risk terrible humiliation if you approached an older sibling.

Gender definition in our country, from the Industrial Revolution to the 1970s when the women's movement shook things up a bit, placed the boys and girls firmly in different camps. Many adults today—certain those I interviewed for this book—feel that being a boy in a family gave them certain privileges and a good deal of freedom; being a girl in the same family saddled you with expectations to be nice, be accommodating, get your brother a sandwich, and clean up after him.

Any whiff of sexuality in a teenage girl of the last generation was usually squelched by her overzealous parents. Dampen it, hide it, bury it, do anything at all but show it.

Sex was very often the only thing that siblings didn't discuss. We had to go to friends to share the scraps of information we all had, to show off the forbidden, wonderful, terrible parts of our body. The grownups had to be keeping all this a secret because it was too big, like the atom bomb. Touching ourselves clearly would set off the detonation.

One day, when we started masturbating, usually in early puberty, or right around the time some of us had our first partnered sexual experience, we saw the truth. Even if we didn't achieve orgasm, the heightened sense of arousal and amazing pleasure made us understand why grownups wanted to keep this to themselves, far away from our consciousness.

How long did it take to get to the truth? Jack, the concert pianist, was a virgin until he was twenty-one and didn't start masturbating until after he had come with a woman. He was sexually threatened by his mother, a passionate Hungarian who used him as an emotional punching bag. His father, on the other hand, was an uptight, silent Englishman. "I was so confused about my sexual feelings, I thought maybe I was gay, maybe I was nothing. I actually asked a girl in college who was a close friend if she'd teach me to kiss. We bought a bottle of tequila and sat around her apartment all night listening to Pink Floyd and making out. It was great. I felt so much better—that I really liked this, so it made me okay. I'd had nocturnal emissions, and I thought orgasm was something you just dreamed about. When I met my first lover, it took twice, but I finally came. I cried, it was so wonderful. I don't think I really felt comfortable about my sexuality until my father died about five years ago."

How do we get comfortable if we aren't? Sometimes, reading erotic literature or seeing pornographic pictures or movies can make us more self-conscious if we are already skittish about this subject. One way a comfort level can be achieved is by masturbating and finding out what you really like—and what you are like. Another way is to talk about sexual issues in a nonthreatening environment, with a person we know casually, in a public place, for example. When there is nothing at stake, like your self-esteem or your embarrassment about not knowing enough, you can express yourself more freely. This will help enormously when it comes to sharing information with those who know even less than you do, like your children.

It's easier when you have help. Maybe you can broach the issue of Kegel exercises with your adolescent daughter while your partner tackles the nitty-gritty of condom selection with your son or daughter. And if both of you feel totally inept in this area, it is a very good idea to solicit the aid of your school guidance counselor or nurse, or a really wonderful teacher who can be a confidant to your kids. They may listen to an authority figure who isn't Mom or Dad. You might also try to find a fabulous adolescent pediatrician or family doctor through referrals from friends or other medical professionals. Any doctor you choose for your child must have an open-door policy when it comes to dealing with and discussing difficult issues.

How to Talk Emotionally to Boys as Well as Girls

We would all like to imagine that we treat our boy children and girl children the same, but it ain't so, not by a long shot. From day one, boys are handled more, girls are talked to more. And by the age of four, girls are already being socialized to be more emotional than boys.

In studies comparing parent–child conversations, particularly about past events, mothers and fathers both discussed feelings with girls more than they did with their boys. They used more emotional words that covered a great range of emotion. Interestingly enough, they talked about sadness more with daughters, and about anger more with sons.

No wonder, by the time these kids are teens, the girls among them are hooked on "relationships," whereas the boys are busy with activities and achievement. It's bred in the bone, and reinforced over and over again in society.

But look what our boys are missing—if talking about our experiences and others' has validity, it is because we attribute a feeling state to what has happened to us.

By teaching children to look at themselves in the midst of a scary or wonderful or mind-boggling event, we allow them to interpret and evaluate their reactions at the time and give them space to think about their consequences later on. If we are responsible enough to teach our four-year-old boy to examine his feelings when he pushes another child down in the playground, we may be guiding him away from sexual harassment in his teen years. When we show our girls how to stand up for themselves and acknowledge their anger at being pushed, we can keep them from becoming victims. By encouraging both of them to talk about the event, we can foster good communication and break down some of the crumbling old edifices of the eternal struggle.

It is important to make your child aware of sexual differences in people—male and female, child and adult, heterosexual and homosexual. Be sure you present your picture without too many negatives and positives. If your children use slang and label people as "faggot" or "dyke," explain why these words are unfair and unkind. You might talk about some friends of yours who live a different lifestyle or have a different sexual orientation. If your kids make fun of older people having sex, tell them that grandma and grandpa undoubtedly have a sexual relationship, since sex is something we can all enjoy until the day we die.

Keep an Open-Door Policy

You don't have to drag up big subjects at dinnertime because you think it's good for everyone to dig into their interpersonal skills along with their mashed potatoes. It can be acutely annoying for children of any age to find their parents lecturing about issues that seemed to appear from nowhere.

You can, however, establish a feeling with your kids that it's okay for them to come to you with anything, whether it's the fact that your daughter tore her best dress and didn't tell you until right before your parents' fiftieth wedding anniversary, or questions about God and the devil. If they know that you aren't going to chastise them or make fun of them, they'll have enough trust in you to broach difficult topics. And particularly if you do this at a young age, when they are more inclined to think that Mom and Dad rule the world, they will approach you for advice when they're older and their rose-colored glasses have fallen off.

You may find that your children are not direct, maybe because they're still testing how deeply they can trust you. They may dance around the issues, so you must develop excellent listening skills to understand just exactly what they're saying. If your fourteen-year-old daughter tells you that a friend of hers got pregnant and is going to be thrown out of school, she may really be saying that she is considering beginning a sexual relationship with a boy and is nervous about losing your love and respect.

To find out the real nature of her comment, you have to first listen to what she's saying and, then, be accepting of the situation she's presented. You might say, "It's terrible that the school wouldn't support her. Are her parents behind her? What about the father of the baby? Are they still seeing each other? Sounds like she could really use a loving partner right now."

By keeping the door—and your mind—open, you may find out what's really bugging her. This doesn't mean that when she tells you she's decided to sleep with her boyfriend, that you necessarily have to congratulate her and go out to buy her condoms and Koromex jelly for her diaphragm. You can voice your opinions as long as you keep in touch with what she's going through and don't shut her out.

If you come up with cop-out phrases like "you're too young," or "you can get AIDS," or "we don't know his family," you will certainly turn your child against you, and either turn her against sex as well or drive her right into a lot of acting-out behavior. What you might say instead is, "I can see how much you care about this person, and being physical together is one way of expressing how you feel. But have you two thought about doing other physical things together first, like massage or bathing or mutual masturbation? Until you've had an ongoing relationship for at least six months, you can't know how you'll react."

This kind of talk will provoke an argument, but it will plant certain seeds that need to grow. It will only be afterwards, in the privacy of their own consciences, that your children may be able to take in all the relevant concerns: getting attached to someone who might not be around in a month, risking pregnancy or HIV disease, risking the censure of classmates or other adults, and losing virginity (if that is still an issue for any kid today).

The open-door policy is even more vital for younger children. A five-year-old who wants to know why Mrs. Thomas is so fat in the middle or an eleven-year-old who wants to know why his penis is erect when he wakes up in the morning, has to be given permission to express all the confusions and curiosity of his or her age. Don't think you have to have all the answers: you're not a teacher or a sex therapist, you're a parent. If you don't know, say that's a good question and you'll have to find out. And then *find out*.

Open the door, just an inch. The kids will do the rest.

Learn What They Know, Don't Know and Are Scared to Death of

Kids have enormous numbers of sources of misinformation these days, starting with TV, going on to friends, school, overheard conversations and coming back to TV. It will be hard for you to beat all these other sources to the draw when it comes to imparting the real facts, figures and feelings.

Don't pry or lecture, but listen first, and ask questions when you don't understand their concerns. A good way of working with your child when you're in the midst of a heavy-duty discussion is to throw out a few common misconceptions or wrongheaded ideas and see if they fly. Ask your kids what they think of the following: "Have sex and you can die from AIDS" or "Lots of kids have babies in high school—their moms take care of them when they're busy" or "Boys should just try to get whatever they can out of girls—it's cool."

These provocative statements will start conversations, and you can supply corrections as you go. Then check back. Ask, was that what you wanted to know?

Your child should feel that if something comes up that is too terrifying or embarrassing to discuss with you, that there's someone else around he or she can trust. Give your child permission to take problems, such as STDs or pregnancy or date rape or drug abuse, to a doctor or counselor. Let him or her know that no parental consent is needed to be tested or treated for any illness. By giving away some of your power to another adult, you may get it back doubled in love and respect from your child.

How Much Do They Learn in School?

Nobody is really thrilled about handling the touchy issue of kids and sex in school. Teachers cringe; administrators smile nervously and look away. Most states currently have some sort of HIV/AIDS awareness-and-prevention requirement in the school systems, but only about half the states in this country are mandated to teach family life education, an expansion of the courses we knew as hygiene, sex ed and civics, all rolled into one.

Actually, family life, if taught properly, is a preparation for being a really terrific human being who can, in fact, do unto others as she would have others do unto her. If taught badly, it can create havoc in a young mind struggling for self-recognition and confidence about dealings with others.

At any rate, this curriculum is presented—albeit briefly—in the great majority of schools around the country, if the parents and religious groups don't protest too much. In grades K to 2, the children are taught a lot about keeping clean and germs and family interaction. They learn about their internal organs and their emotions and feelings. By grade 3, they are up to body parts, and in fourth grade, they get a little on genetics and heredity. In fifth and sixth grade, they start the tough stuff about adolescent changes and safer sex.

Then they reach puberty and school officials get very anxious. According to the Alan Guttmacher Institute, America's high schools offer only 6.5 hours of sex education per year. Middle schools teach even less.

The topics are listed in order by the typical amount of coverage given:

- Healthy child development (e.g., body parts, puberty)
- Self-esteem and universal values
- HIV/AIDS
- Pregnancy and reproduction
- Decision-making skills
- Responsible personal behavior (e.g., abstinence, moral value system)
- Behavioral skills (e.g., refusal skills, communicating about sex)
- Risks/dangers of premature sex (e.g., teen pregnancy)
- Sex in society (e.g., media messages)
- Sexually transmitted diseases (STDs)
- Sexual violence (date, acquaintance, and stranger rape; sex abuse)
- Contraception and condoms

- Sexual orientation (homosexuality, bisexuality, and heterosexuality)
- Masturbation
- Abortion/choice
- Sexual pleasure
- Sexual expression without risk ("outercourse," necking, mutual masturbation).

See how far down on the list you have to go to get up to pleasure and sexual expression? Incredible that anyone would like sex after being warned through the years about all the various hassles (from mildly annoying to life-threatening) you have to go through to be a sexual person. It is to be expected, of course, that teachers fear the administration and parental censure if they promote the healthful or rewarding aspects of human sexuality. I served on a curriculum revision committee in my own township where supposedly enlightened parents nearly came to blows over what they wanted their children to learn and how they wanted the material presented. Inform kids that sex is healthful and fun and not just for reproduction? Scandalous! Show kids that even if their desires and fantasies are different from the mainstream, that's okay? Never! Give kids the emotional tools to protect themselves and their partners? Unheard of!

Do teachers just teach the facts, or do they work on feelings? Do teachers aim for the "right" answer in class, or do they provide a forum for open discussion where any idea is acceptable to try out? Do they feel okay enough with the subject matter to offer it in a non-biased manner? Whew! Who knows? You'd have to be a fly on the wall in your kids' classrooms through the years to hear how this heady stuff is presented. You can add your two cents by making an appointment with the teacher or guidance counselor in charge of this program, finding out what's going on, and offering your support and encouragement. If we champion our teachers for doing this difficult work, they will be cheered on to continue it.

The most significant part of family life education that is most often ignored is that teachers are there to present the issues and facts, *not* to put forth their own values and ethical beliefs. That's for the family to do. You've got to find out what your school is teaching and then, amplify the ideas, say what you really feel about sex and sexuality. Your values will shape your child's thinking for years to come, but you don't want to sock him with such rigid beliefs that he won't have room to develop some of his own when the time is right. But if you abdicate responsibility for this job, your child is getting only half an education.

Simpler Is Better: Talking to Young Children

Children are naturally comfortable in their bodies. Watch a baby roll around on a carpet, sticking her toes in her mouth; watch a toddler jump up and down endlessly on a mattress, screaming with delight; and you'll see what they've got that you've lost. But parents often squelch this fabulous feeling by giving off messages, subtle and direct, that it's not great to be *too* comfortable.

When we indicate body parts to our little ones, statistics show that we name "elbows, toes, knees, armpits" many more times and with much more assurance in our voices than we do "vulva, vagina, penis, anus"—if in fact we name those parts at all. When children want to know what those areas down below are called, we often come up with euphemisms that stick. (And if we don't, the grandparents, baby-sitters, and other children in the neighborhood will do it.)

Give your girls and boys mirrors so they can see not just their faces, but all their parts. Teach them to enjoy exploration. If you notice your toddler rubbing and squeezing his or her genitals, it's important to point out that this activity is wonderful and feels very good, but it should be kept private, because touching ourselves this way is a very personal thing we don't share with others until we're much older. Emphasize that Mom and Dad need their privacy too, for the same reasons.

Be tender with your child's sense of emotional comfort, as well. By holding and caressing your child and expressing your love verbally at the same time, you are telling him or her that touch and feelings are linked.

Parents are often panic-stricken when they get the first question that will surely lead to an embarrassing answer, whether it's "Why don't I have a penis?" or "Does the baby come out the same place as my poop?" At the beginning, you need go no further than the basic information. The answer to the first question is "Because you're a girl and girls have vulvas instead of penises," and the answer to the second is "No, you have another hole in front of the anus where the bowels come out, and that vaginal opening is where the baby comes out."

Naming names is essential. Small children need small answers. They have to know first what something is called, and second, what it does. That's all. When they're ready to ask bigger questions, we can tackle them.

Be concrete. Use simple words. Check on what you've done by asking, "have I answered your question?" or "Is there anything else you want to know?" Do it with humor and good grace, and you'll be fine.

How to Talk About Sex to School-Age Children

When your children are older, there are many influences on their thinking and their perception of the information they've been given, whether on the street or in a classroom. From the ages of about seven to eleven, it's how you say it, rather than what you say, that makes a difference.

Don't fudge it. Children know when you're skirting an issue or not really at ease with what you're giving forth. They already have the basics, so it's just spinning your wheels to go over the same factual territory about the differences between boys and girls and the plumbing inside. Dull. No kid wants to hear it again, and you'll turn them right off if you persist.

What they want now is emotions. How you feel about liking someone, wanting to touch someone, wanting to be intimate, is a lot more relevant to a school-age child. And what's essential, as you impart the message that touch is great and good (which they should have had from you since birth if you've been hugging, kissing, and holding them), is that *sexual* touch is fraught with physical and emotional complications that children are not ready to handle. Rather than giving the big fear lecture to scare them into abstinence, you want to paint a deeply rewarding but ultimately over-their-heads picture of what it's going to be like.

You do want younger kids to wait. Overstimulation is scary for a child—they just don't know how to handle the huge emotional upheaval that comes along with expressing their sexuality. It's not just that you can get HIV disease from "going all the way," it's that you can find yourself incapable of handling the tears and loss of self-esteem and judgment of your peers if your relationship falls apart. It's that the new exploration of your body by another may be overwhelming to a kid and feel more like a violation of space and invasion of privacy than true intimacy. You want to get across the idea that childhood is for getting to like and understand yourself well enough so that when you're older you can express this to another and receive the same back.

Children will be curious about how bodies fit together, but they are also curious about relationships. You may have some very fixed attitudes about "no sex until marriage" or "don't let anyone touch you until you're sure you love them." Understand, however, that these attitudes have screwed up generations of individuals. Of course there is a tendency in each one of us parents to want to keep our children in a bubble, safe from the thorns and prickles of real life, but it can't be done. We have to acknowledge that they are going to experiment (as we did), and they will be hurt by those they never should have slept with and they will pine for those who will never want to sleep with them.

Listen to their concerns and voice your own. Then let all this stuff percolate for a while. They will make mistakes (as we did), but with your support, they will make good decisions as well.

How to Talk and Listen to Your Teens

Nearly half of the children in this country over the age of twelve are sexually active. By the age of eighteen, 75 percent of males and 60 percent of females have had intercourse. However busy they may be *doing* it, it is very difficult to get them to *talk* about it. Why? Because they know all about it—they know everything—and don't have to discuss it. They are inflicted with the four I's—they are invincible, immortal, immune, and infertile—so of course nothing can happen to them. Whether you are discussing sex with a ghetto kid, a suburban kid, or a Park Avenue kid, you never get anywhere if you tell them not to do what they intend to do. Their hormones are raging, they are determined to break with old family structures and become independent, and they have some very substantial opinions of their own, formed through influence of family, school, friends, media, religious organizations, and personal philosophy.

Most teens, unless they come from a very open household, won't bring up the subject at all. The ball is in your camp when you see the time is right. A newscast about a rape case, a close friend with HIV, an aunt whose boyfriend just ran out on her, a friend whose daughter is pregnant, may offer ample opportunity to talk about issues without getting personal.

By all means, stay away from judgments and hold the guilt. Whatever you offer of your own should reward self-esteem and personal decision-making skills. Don't use yourself as an example— most teens don't believe their parents have a sex life anyway, and the great majority would think it's a big hoot to hear about your wild times way back when. So stay away from self-congratulatory stories ("how I learned from my mistakes and got wiser and mellower") and instead, learn how to listen, *really listen* to them.

To change any behavior, new messages have to be internalized. The worth of whatever values you are trying to inculcate in your kids has to make sense. Most of us fight the system before learning how to change it or fit ourselves inside it. Sometimes, we have to do some pretty drastic maneuvers to vault the impenetrable wall life sets up for us before we can come over to the other side. This may mean that your children have to go through their own trial by fire, and you are not allowed to throw water on the conflagration. But you can help them by keeping that door, and your mind, open.

If your teen asks you about sex, ask back. Test the emotional waters by finding out the following:

- Are you ready to accept a physical and emotional change in yourself, the sense of being different from many of your peers?
- Are you ready to accept a "reputation" if anyone finds out?
- Are you ready for rejection when the affair ends?
- Are you ready for the mental distraction of maintaining this intense emotional relationship which may take you away from other friends and pursuits?
- Are you ready to take risks, physical and emotional, that include STDs, pregnancy, and depression?

As your teenager becomes more comfortable discussing some of this with you, it may be possible to work in the fact that you love her and want to make sure she doesn't hurt herself too badly. Positive risk-taking is necessary for growth, but not negative risk taking. Just because your child is pressured socially to do like everyone on the TV sitcoms does, is no reason to jump into bed.

And for teens, usually, there isn't any bed. The backseat of a car, a less than secluded corner of a parking lot, a strip of beach all provide exciting but less than optimal situations for first sexual encounters. Talk about furtive! Talk about hurried! They could be discovered and uncovered at any moment. Most kids can't surrender freely with all these constraints, and a bad first experience can sour the taste for a long time to come—*if* they can come.

Teens have sexual encounters for many reasons: to earn love, comfort, money, to get physical relief, to exert power, because they're bored, because their friends do it, because it's fun, because they can't say no, because they're out to prove that they're very masculine or very feminine, because they're under the influence of drugs or alcohol. Or because they want to get back at you in the worst way.

Forget, for a moment, your desire to keep your children safe and sound, and concentrate on getting them to clarify their own thinking on this issue. If they know their reasons before they act, they can evaluate their behavior. They may even be able to postpone or change the nature of what they do because of what they feel.

Do problem-solving exercises with your teens. Let them seriously consider the ramifications of their actions—on themselves, their families and their potential lovers. In this way, they can develop a responsible value system—not yours, not society's, but their very own.

What Can You Do to Protect Your Child from a Teen Pregnancy?

Teen pregnancy is a terrifying prospect. It's frightening for the child having the baby and it's frightening for the parents of that child. Although the number of teens who are diagnosed HIV positive is growing at an alarming rate, a far more present danger is that your son or daughter will come home and inform you that he or she is about to become a parent.

When babies have babies, it is detrimental to our society. But even worse is the way teen pregnancy can wreak havoc with so many lives in one family.

How does it happen in this climate where condoms and spermicidal agents are available in every supermarket and drugstore? We may say that some teenagers are unlucky, and their contraception fails—condoms, diaphragms, and even the pill and IUD can occasionally fall down on the job. But in most cases, the child who becomes pregnant does not know how to use contraception effectively, has been doing some magical thinking about how "getting knocked up" only happens to other people, or has been conned into thinking that sex is too beautiful to spoil with pausing to be careful. It happens because we've been careful about teaching teens the facts, but completely remiss about making abstract facts into real, crucial, responsible actions.

The problems of teen pregnancy are too numerous:

- Does the couple intend to keep the baby? How can they finish school and start a meaningful type of work?

- Does the couple intend to have an abortion? Who will they ask to help them in this decision? Who will pay for it?

- Is the pregnant girl going it alone? Has she been abandoned by the one person (the father of her child) she thought she could trust?

- Does she feel like a pariah at school? Will anyone—boys or girls—even want to spend time with her?

- Does she feel like a pariah at home? Will her parents and siblings reject her?

- Will she tell an authority figure in time to have a safe abortion?

- Will she have the proper resources to get adequate prenatal care should she decide to keep the baby?

- Will she be mature enough to give up the baby for adoption to a family who might be able to give the child a better life?

- Will she be able to manage (along with her parents, grandparents, or other relatives) taking care of a child and getting on with her own life?

- Is the young man who fathered the child ready to accept his responsibility, or is he turning it back on the girl, claiming "she must have slept around"?

- Is the young man feeling alienated from his friends and family, unsure of how he can take care of a new family of his own?

Teenagers get pregnant on purpose or "by accident" for many reasons—to assert their independence or get even with parents, to snare a desirable mate, or to feel a type of love they've never known. Many girls say that they desperately desire the sense of unconditional love they believe they will have from a tiny infant. Yet they have no comprehension, before the child comes into the world, of the type of responsibilities—personal, financial, emotional, social— they will have to shoulder in order to bring up a child. Nor do they have any way of gauging their own anger and frustration with a newborn who needs round-the-clock attention. The phenomenon of child mothers abandoning or severely injuring their new babies is a terrifyingly common one.

Make sure your child know what having a baby is all about. The American Red Cross offers excellent baby-sitting courses for girls from ten to eighteen that will give just a hint of what life after birth might be like.

Helping Your Child to Gain Social Intelligence

Think about all the ways in which we are smart. Some of us are great with verbal skills, or math, some have an innate ability to listen to a tune and write a harmony for it. Some people have a great kinesthetic sense—movement speaks in their bodies, and they can copy anyone else's movement perfectly. And some of us are wonderful athletes, able to leap tall hurdles at a single bound, able to aim just right as we catch and throw.

But there is also a social intelligence (described by Howard Gardner in his excellent book, *Frames of Mind*) that allows us to interact with others. No one bothers to foster this intelligence, in school or out of it. Yet unless we are socially savvy, how can we be sexually responsible? How can we know just what it is about another person that attracts us or turns us off?

Give your children the gift of learning this about themselves: that they will only find that illusory quality we call love when they can really pick up on their capacity to express their touch, to communicate their feelings, and to give of themselves freely to a friend of either sex. This is stuff you don't learn from a book. And as a parent, you can be the guide to steer them toward the life experience they need to hone their social and sexual smarts.

Give Your Children the Passion of Your Ideas

Please talk about real feelings with your children. Don't just talk—*feel* with them. This has to be one of the best preparations you can give for the rest of your child's life. When your kids can delve deep into themselves with you as their guide, they can figure out what their feelings really are, get a bead on what to do with them, and understand that other people may have feelings that don't necessarily coincide with theirs. Respect for a partner in a sexual relationship is so essential that it bears some repetition here.

I am horrified by the rampant sexual attacks that go on in junior and senior high schools around the country. Boys in packs prowl hallways and locker rooms to attack their female classmates (so far, girls have not attacked boys, but who knows when those demanding justice and revenge may turn the tables). Urban ghetto populations have seen the advent of "whirlpooling," which takes place in public pools in the summer. Boys gang up forming a circle and hold onto each others' shoulders as they trawl for female victims. They surround these girls (who may not be helpless, but are simply outnumbered and vulnerable in the water where they can't run away), and, chanting rap slogans that tend to denigrate women, they attack. Imagine how humiliating and debasing it must be to have your bathing suit torn off and to be sexually molested by a gang. Is it worse if you've been friends with your attackers? If you've done school projects together and gone on class trips together? And yet, in the context of the pool, you are a hunted animal.

It's not just in the inner city that this takes place. Young people who grow up not being taught that they must pay attention to someone else's needs and wants continue harassing others as adults. Would sexual harassment on campuses and in businesses be such an issue if we talked to our kids about their sexuality and made them responsible for it? I doubt it.

A boy whose parents never told him how raging hormones would make him forget the world and feel justified in getting immediate gratification is likely to keep hammering away at a girlfriend who is possibly interested in kissing, but no more. A girl whose parents have never clarified the confusion she feels between wanting to be stroked and held and the guilt of giving away her "cherry" is not going to be straight with a boy when she starts making out, never intending to complete the act of intercourse. These two could end up in a date-rape situation because they can't talk about what's really going on. She isn't saying no, she doesn't want him, because she does. He isn't saying that he can be satisfied with a little kissing and petting, and afterward he'll masturbate while she watches (or doesn't watch, if that's her preference), because nobody ever mentioned this was a viable alternative.

Consensual sex among young people is possible only if they learn to be straight with one another. And where else would they learn that but back home, under their parents' roof? If teens understood how much was involved in the brief act of intercourse—physically, emotionally, psychically, socially, morally—they would abstain far more than they are currently doing. This doesn't mean they would be depriving their sexual drives in any way—please reread Chapter Five if you have any doubts as to other pleasurable activities that can be substituted for intercourse.

If you are a caring parent, and you can remember your own miseducation, you will have the compassion to give your kids the easy comfort with masturbation, homosexuality, and even lack of interest in partners of either sex. Children are thirsty sponges; they soak up life experience and wring out just those elements that seem to make the most sense. Even if you have acute pangs about a son who prefers dance class to football practice, or a daughter who wants to starve herself so she'll look beautiful for the next available suitor, open yourself to the idea that anything is possible. The gay aspect may pass, or it may be in the process of solidifying itself. The anorexia may be transitory, or it may be working its way into a serious pattern of illness. But you will only find out if you stop, look, and pay attention to your kids' sexual needs.

So let them say the words! Say them out loud together! Listen to them—really listen! Give them the confidence they so rightly deserve about their sexuality and what they want to do with it as they grow up. You will add immeasurably to the future of our planet.

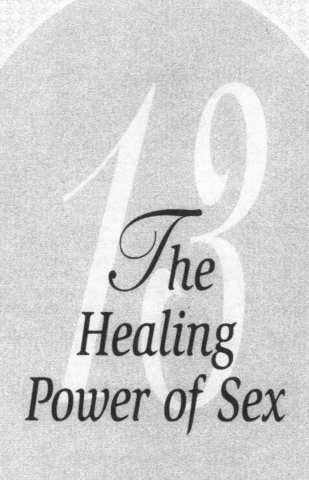

13

The Healing Power of Sex

*I*f you are truly healthy, you are in a state of harmony with yourself and your surroundings. You have to have a sense of proportion throughout all facets of your life—not just one part of it. It won't do you a whole lot of good to have a peak-performance body that you torture with food withdrawal and exercise mania if your soul is not in good shape, if your relationships are falling apart, if you don't like yourself or your living accommodations or your children.

To be really healthy, you have to have it all in balance, not caring so much about any one feature. And if you can achieve that, you can begin to approach what psychologist and personal-growth revolutionary Abram Maslow described as "peak experiences" and what Joseph Campbell termed "following your bliss."

Will your sexuality help you to achieve bliss? How could it not? When you feel just right as a sexual being, everything else you are is in perfect equilibrium. By achieving the potential of your *sexuality*:

- You can express yourself better verbally and nonverbally.
- You can be more creative in your job or avocation.
- You can exert power when you have to.
- You can sit back and learn from a mentor.
- You can have fun.
- Others will gravitate toward you, as though you were a particularly powerful magnet.
- You can feel physically as strong as lightning, as gentle as a mild rain.

By pursuing only your *sex* potential:

- You will feel desperate to look "right"—like a perfect "10."
- You may grasp at others greedily instead of attracting them.
- You may be victimized by others in your attempt to make yourself likable.

- You may be perceived as manipulative instead of reciprocal in your relationships.
- You may exploit others for your pleasure.

You will be totally out of balance, out of sync with yourself and your environment.

Beyond Sexual Release

Let us say you could never have sex again, either with yourself or with another person. Is that a crippling thought? A terrifying one? Or would it fill you with relief?

If you could never have sex again, what would you substitute for it? Many people interviewed for this book said that they would use their other appetites instead. One woman answered immediately, "I'd eat chocolate while riding a horse." Food was a big first answer, followed by music, art, exercise and good friends. One man said he would spend his time watching old black-and-white movies, vicariously being Cary Grant or Clark Gable—whom you never saw actually making love on screen anyway. Several individuals said they would become much more productive mentally, taking unused sexual power from their body and channeling it to the life of the mind and soul.

When you think of sex as a big buildup and then a delirious release, you are shortchanging yourself. For some, it takes just a few seconds to build up to an orgasm and "get off." And at the end of that brief explosive excursion, you feel depleted, tired, drained. When you're so intent on zooming to the heights, you never bother to learn about how to float outward into other realms instead of crashing to the depths afterward.

When you eliminate the need for a quick release, or a fast fix or an immediate solution, you prolong the pleasure. You give yourself and your partner the gift of time.

Maybe, then, if you couldn't *have* sex, you would *be sexual*. You would expand your attractiveness from the body to the spirit; you would push past the barriers of needing another person to fulfill your body's destiny and make yourself responsible for your own pleasure. You would become fully creative and each thing you did, each thought you had, would be an orgasm of expression.

Luckily, for most of us, this scenario will never have to take place. We can be sexual and have sex until the day we die, if we want to.

How Does Your Sexuality Translate into Good Health?

Imagine a large power generator, churning out millions of megawatts each day and night, never ceasing. It could light up a city; it could heat every residence and business; it could provide enough sustenance for crops to grow and flourish.

Your body is exactly like a generator, using sexuality for fuel. But you must know how to turn it on and how to channel this extraordinary energy. Many individuals interviewed for this book told me that they were confused and overwhelmed by the reactions they and others had to their sexual feelings.

"I'm like a caged animal sometimes, wanting it so badly, and then when it's released, I turn into this wild banshee, my body out of control, my brain blanking out. It's frightening to my husband," a woman in midlife said. She is troubled by the way her sexuality takes over; but when she learns enough about herself to use this force constructively, she will be in charge. Her passion, her spontaneous release, her ability to relax and let the energy move her, her ability to communicate (even when the outcome seems frightening to her partner), her willingness to be a sexual creature no matter how animalistic and primitive she feels, all show that she's on the right healing course.

How can we use our sexual energy to be more creative, feel better, look better, be better?

- Pleasure your body and mind every day. This means eating and exercising well, wearing clothing that feels good on your skin, enjoying a languid bath or invigorating shower.
- Recognize your sexual feelings, never ignore them.
- Try to imagine pushing your physical urge upward, letting it course through the body to the heart and head.
- Make a connection between your bodily hunger and yearning and a particular goal in everyday life that you wish to accom-

plish. There are parallels between your appetite for another person and your desire to learn to play a musical instrument, for example.

How have you perceived your sexuality in the past?

- Have you used it for power over a partner?
- Have you used it as a way to get attention or affection?
- Have you seen it as a chore that must be accomplished?
- Has it offered a respite from boredom?
- Have you seen it as a means to some other end?
- Has it been a way for you to buoy up your self-esteem?

If you are truly committed to using your sexuality outside the scope of physical intercourse, you must revise your vision of what sexuality means to you. There are far more beneficial ways to gain these than "being sexy," and it will take some doing to downplay your craving for bodily contact or approval and channel it toward productive daily activity. But you can do it, and will over time if you are patient with yourself and your partners.

How to Make Your Old Lover into Someone New

We are aroused in different ways and for different reasons. Some of us tend to like comfort with our sex, and the rituals we set up with a partner over time lull us into the security of knowing we will always be well loved in this way.

But most individuals, particularly those who've been partnered with one other individual for many years—heterosexual or homosexual—get that itch. Our fantasies often revolve around others—if I were with him or her, what could I do? Where could we do it? How would it feel? The unknown in the land of sex is a powerful lure because it challenges us to dare to be different, to explore uncharted realms that may seem scary and overwhelming.

Just a few decades ago, it was hip to have many partners, multiple partners. To our sorrow, we realized that spreading the bounty has opened a Pandora's box of infection and death. Today, it is the irresponsible, immature adult who jumps from bed to bed—not only because of the many sexually transmitted diseases but because it implies that the individual has no spine, no stick-to-itiveness. And our basically American credo is "Stay with the job until it's done right." Divorce isn't cool anymore because it means you break up your family, you and your ex have to deal with your existential aloneness, and you're in the dangerous marketplace once more. Living with a person of the opposite sex and then discovering that you are really attracted to a person of your own sex is difficult because society can't figure you out and will probably shun you, and possibly your children, for your choice. Adultery is a hard choice because it implies you can't put all your eggs in one basket, pledging allegiance to one individual in one marriage for time immemorial.

But there are some real loopholes in our adherence to strict monogamy. Those people who have high scores on the sex, love, and marriage scale developed by researchers in a 1986 study showed that people who really bought into this romantic idea of one long-term partner tended to restrict themselves in their sexual expression.

Their attitudes about gender orientation were fixed ("Men are men, women are women, and anything in between is wrong."), they had little premarital experience and had more guilt in relation to doing anything, even going to the movies with a friend, that was not exclusive in their relationship. Their levels of jealousy were high; their ability to pursue activities and interests that they did not share with their partner was low. If love of a single partner keeps you bound up so tightly, no wonder you get bored and itchy. No wonder so many couples end up in the offices of marriage counselors and sex therapists, demanding their rights, or complaining about lack of compatibility.

What would be ideal is to keep the structure and closeness of a long-term partnership and give it variety and freedom. This is very difficult to do. In centuries past, when people didn't live so long (and therefore couldn't be married to one person for so long), and where exclusivity in a sexual relationship was necessary for the preservation of the tribe, monogamy had a true purpose. In today's world, where we may live beyond our centennials, what makes much more sense is serial commitments (one enduring relationship for a period of years, and then the next, and then the next).

But if you feel committed to one person for the long run, what you must do is learn to split your one partner into many while at the same time consolidating that single relationship you have forged.

One way to change the person you are with in your imagination is to see him or her as a descendant in a great line of your sexuality. Everything you have been is a part of what you are sexually. This includes the people in the past that you have loved well. You can't recreate with your current lover what you had with someone else, but it is possible to recapture that long-ago wonder and freedom of expression. Allow the spirits of all your past relationships into your bedroom now and let them help you feel joy in the present. Your current partner is the culmination of these others in your experience, and your feelings and your physical potential with this person can rise to be the highest they've ever been.

Avoiding Ruts and Habits

If you've been with someone a long time, it's natural to fall into routines. These are nice because they give you a sense of continuity with one another, but they get boring and can lead to sexual burnout. To make your old lover into someone new, you would have to behave as though you had never touched before. Impossible, really. What you can do, however, is to shift the ground under your feet and make yourselves accommodate to the change around you.

Leading and Following

Don't be a Sleeping Beauty or a Sir Galahad. They waited, as so many mythological characters do, to let the more aggressive partner make all the moves. We don't know what happened to these innocents afterward, but I would bet that they allowed their partners to initiate sex most of the time, putting the other person in charge of all the sexual decisions. This is not the hallmark of a sexually mature couple.

To gain balance in your life, you must be an equal partner. When you become aware of who usually makes the sexual decisions, and how, it will be easier to reciprocate. You have to wake up and respond, whether that response is, "I don't want to right now" or "That's a great idea." This will make it easier to decide that you feel sexual and want to act on it.

Balancing Pleasure Between You

Some like coffee, some like tea. You don't always get a partner who agrees with everything, whether it's a business decision or whether it's their turn to change the catbox. This is also true in bed. What really turns one person on may leave the other cold. You have to talk about it so that you get your goodies too, but not all the time.

Even mature sexual couples disagree on frequency, activity, and who should be on top. This is not an activity that requires a completely united front. You may think you're pleasing your partner by agreeing to something that makes you uncomfortable, but in the long run, faking an orgasm or having sex in order to make up after a fight is a mistake. Experimenting with another form of pleasure you aren't sure about may be an interesting idea that will restore balance—just be sure that if you don't like the bondage or the anal sex, you say so.

Playacting

We are not always what we seem. It can be neat in sex to try on different roles. You may never use foul language in your everyday life, but you may find yourself moved to say, "I love fucking you," in bed. You may be a cynical, streetwise, urban tough guy, but showering your mate with flowers and poetry may feel nice for a change. Some couples actually dress in costume for sex, and of course the Eastern traditions (see below) recommend the ritual of presexual enticement, using fans, scarves, drapes and flowers arranged in a certain veiled and mysterious manner. You are entering a country of unknown adventures, sights and sounds. So pretending to be an animal or a spy or a cowboy or a *femme* or *homme fatale* is perfectly right.

Play with your sex. Dress it up and take it on the town.

Keep Each Sexual Encounter in Its Own Moment

The only time you have together is now. There is no purpose in imagining what an encounter will be like, or what you want to make happen, because undoubtedly it won't, and you'll end up disappointed. Many people tell me that the anticipation of sex is often greater than the reward, and the reason is that they have some intention or agenda to accomplish.

Whatever happens is okay—if you went to bed expecting fifty orgasms and didn't come once, or if you really wanted a slow, sensuous massage on cushions on the floor and got a quickie on top of the kitchen table, so be it. Next time, it can all be different. There will be something in each encounter that is thrilling. If you stay in the moment, you will discover its unique wonder.

Creating a Spiritual Bond: Flowing with Your Partner

Think about the French phrase for orgasm: *le petit mort*, which translates as "the little death." Maybe that fainting, swooning, loss of consciousness that comes when we come is something to look forward to, rather than fear.

The meaning of the phrase is not death but liberation. We can pass from the quotidien world to a space and time that is beyond reality. We can fly if we choose to.

When you are sexually intimate with a partner who is there for you completely and without restrictions, the two of you can merge while still retaining your own individuality. Sex can change two individuals into one unit, flowing effortlessly in and out of their own egos. This experience is similar to that known to mystics and religious devotees who reach high levels of consciousness through meditation and prayer.

The flow, as described by psychologist Mihaly Csikszentmihalyi, is a state where you become one with the activity you're involved with—the basketball player is the ball careening through the hoop; the runner is the stream of moving limbs that carry him forward in space; the pianist is the music, pouring out of a passionate mind and heart. Children, of course, are in "the flow" most of the time, dedicating themselves so thoroughly to their play that they can sometimes forget time, space, and their personal boundaries.

We can be like that with a partner as well. When our sense of ourselves as a couple is clear and our focus completely on the pleasure we give and receive, we can blend. This takes the sexual experience higher, out of the realm of body. A.J., a forty-year-old landscape architect, said of her lover, "When we get like this, our essence comes together, we dissolve into each other's energy. We leave our bodies and our souls become integrated, kind of like a force field or a cloud melding with another cloud. There is a purpose to our being together."

How to Get Spiritual in Bed

How do you achieve this lofty state? Some couples offer concrete ways:

- Remove distractions—no radios, kids or phones.
- Stay in the moment—each touch is singularly important in and of itself and need not lead to any other touch.
- Create a focus—watch a candle flame between you.
- Keep your focus, and if it wanders away, bring it back to your pleasure and your partner's.
- Try to see the scene from your partner's perspective.
- Synchronize your breathing together.
- Eliminate boredom—try not kissing or not penetrating during one lovemaking session.

Extending Your Life:
Eastern Thought and the Uses of Touch

In the East, sexuality is assumed to have a deeply spiritual nature. The creation of the world, for the most advanced antique cultures, had to do with the procreative joy inherent in the female element. The Goddess with her fecund vulva and multitiered breasts, her abundant orgiastic pleasure in giving forth life, was the first progenitor.

Spirit is one way we can orient our sexuality because when we are truly sexually in sync with ourselves and our partner, we are lifted up beyond ourselves, past our everyday, mundane life. The

Eastern cultures, be they Indian (the Tantrics) or Chinese (the Taoists) or modern-day practitioners who call this way of being sexual *karezza* believe that sexuality is the primary factor in healing and regenerating the universe. If you can train your body to utilize sexual energy, you can process it into creative, healing energy. Some Taoists believe that you can actually build bone marrow and develop higher brain centers with proper use of your sexual energy.

The practice of *tantra* (which means "weaving") unifies the many parts of the self into a whole—we are not male or female, dark or light, matter or energy, but one higher element that contains everything.

This is a pretty lofty goal for the average person with average sexual goals. But if you allow yourself to consider the possibilities inherent in these practices, you can extend yourself and your sexual experiences. If your highest goal was a simultaneous orgasm with your partner, or becoming multiorgasmic yourself, you may be surprised at the fact that these goals are just beginnings when it comes to "high sex," as Margo Anand calls it in *The Art of Sexual Ecstasy.* You can be much more than a body (or two bodies), striving to give each other momentary pleasure.

Tantric and Taoist sex both require the individual or partners to exert control over their orgasms and for men, over their ejaculation. The Indians and Chinese developed these practices centuries ago, and, although rather arcane and not commonly used, they work if you work at them.

According to the ancient texts, longevity could be extended if a couple was willing to conserve their life energy. Many teachers, from the Chinese to the thinkers who wrote the Bible, advised against wasting precious sperm or eggs which might create new life. Onan was cursed by God because he spilled his seed upon the ground so as not to impregnate his late brother's wife. But the great Chinese masters took this one step further—they were able to bring their partners to ecstasy while never ejaculating. These elderly men would exhaust dozens of young women, stealing their partner's *jing* (or vital energy) with each female orgasm.

In modern Taoist and Tantric practice, the following elements are crucial:

- You must mix your male and female elements. Both partners are dominant and receptive.

- You must be able to relax completely at each stage of your excitement. Instead of building to that crashing crescendo we know so well as the Big O, you must allow the tension you feel as you reach your peak to melt as you calm your inner self and avoid the rush to orgasmic impact.

- You must delay gratification. Even if you lose your erection or your arousal, don't be concerned—the genitals are only one source of stimulation for the higher energy systems of the body, in the heart and the mind.

- You must be able to channel the intense sexual fires you feel "down below" up higher in the body. The Tantrics refer to the seven *chakras* or body centers; the Taoists talk about the *microcosmic orbit,* a circuit of energy that goes up the back and down the front. You are counseled to use "the Big Draw" as you visualize and feel your energy traveling up from your groin to your anus to your spine and at last to the top of the head.

- You must master breathing techniques and muscle control. When you feel you are about to come, you inhale and draw the excitement upward in your body as you clench your PC muscles. This prevents an immediate genital orgasm and yet gives the body a gentle all-over wash of pleasure, a kind of "holistic orgasm," as it were.

- You must gain a sense of your body being a conduit for what is happening in your mind and spirit. When you are with a partner, your desire must transmogrify into a joy at blending or melding with the other. Although a lot of everyday sex is bound up in our ego—in what we want others to think about us and what we think about ourselves—in "high sex," there are no selves. There is just one spirit, one energy, one moment in time that seems to be endless.

It sounds impossible, out of reach, a little hallucinatory, doesn't it? There is no way to give a prescription in this book for easy shortcuts to Tantric or Taoist bliss. The best way to achieve higher sex is to read some books on the subject (see Resource Guide), and ideally, to find a partner who is already on the road you wish to follow.

But will practicing these techniques extend your life? As to how sex really has an impact on longevity, let me propose the following:

you live longer if you are in a deeply committed relationship that you choose not to lose. There are so many cases of people *deciding* when they were going to die, based on a family or life event to which they were looking forward. Anecdotal evidence indicates that people sometimes stick around because they feel needed and wanted, and they think that their partner would never survive without them.

Unraveling the Paradox of Good and Bad Sex

If sex is such a beneficial experience, why does it create so many problems? Why is there incest and rape and pornography; why are there sexually transmitted diseases? Why does the deadly HIV virus spread from one individual to another during the sexual act?

As I've said throughout this book, our sexuality is a multifaceted, complex gift. When we don't know how to use it, it can be extremely dangerous. In all fairy tales, when the heroine or hero is handed those ubiquitous three wishes, there is a caveat attached. *Something awful will happen if you don't chose wisely.* And no one ever uses his or her magic wishes properly because they are too greedy, asking for everything and giving nothing in return.

Because we seem to be constitutionally unable to look at the dark side before plunging ahead in the light, we neglect the simplest rule of using our sexuality well: respect and care for your partner as you do yourself.

Sex is power. When it is used in anger, atrocities like the rape of thousands of Bosnian women occur, and sexual experimentation and torture such as that used by the Nazis and the military regimes in South America and elsewhere. Children are destroyed by parents and other adults when sex is used as punishment, and adults are unnaturally stimulated by snuff porn videos and tapes that show people killing victims during sexual acts.

Sex is chemical. When you mix chemicals in a test tube, you may get a wonderful new combination, or you may get an explosive. Knowing what you're doing takes time. You have to mix the elements carefully for every experiment, and in the sexual realm, this means preparing for an encounter with safety precautions in place. Lovers must honor each other with safer sex and good hygiene and an open, caring mental attitude.

Sex provokes the deepest human feelings, among them jealousy and desperation. When we feel "stuck" in a relationship, we can't breathe, we can't feel comfortable in our own skins. One radical solution might be to expand the idea of monogamy, which has caused so much grief for so many. What about a marriage or partnership that is completely flexible and allows adjunct relationships with members of both sexes?

My belief is that we should have the opportunity to share our sexuality with more than one partner, because we express ourselves so differently with different people. We can be one person to a lifetime partner; we can be someone else with a longtime friend with whom we share sexual intimacies; we can be a totally new person with a new lover.

Sex requires a delicate balance of passion and judgment. If we could take sex out of dark corners and make condoms as accessible and commonplace as chewing gum, if we could take the onus off pre- and extramarital sex and require lessons in the pleasures of the body along with geometry and literature, the horrors of sexual abuse would never take place. Those of us who care about this precious ability all humans possess must be the front-runners. We can't have healthy sex until our fitness rating for thinking about sex is sufficiently high. Those who can't handle it must be taught, and if they cannot be taught, they must be restrained.

How You Can Use
the Healing Energy of Sex

We can undercut the violence in our society. When you think about the affectional bonds that draw us into a family, into a love relationship, into a sexual union, you can understand more clearly what we humans can be when we're functioning at our very best. Those who live at the outskirts of our culture—the criminal, the psychotic, the sociopath, the affectless—these people are totally lacking in sexuality, regardless of how much sex they may have. With certain species of chimpanzees, the free-mating males and females take care of one another and their offspring. They may have many partners, but they have one community. And that, ideally, is how we should all be.

Developmental neuropsychologist and cross-cultural psychologist James W. Prescott has shown that the more physical affection shown to infants and the less repressive the sexual taboos in a society, the lower is the incidence of adult physical violence, crime, and warfare. In cultures where babies are carried and cuddled, where they are weaned relatively late, where the people have little stake in displays of individual wealth and where premarital and extramarital sexuality are tolerated, there tends to be more harmony in the entire community. People are peaceful when their pleasure in one another isn't founded in domination and power struggles. If we are to become truly aware individuals, we must take advantage of the *great value of our sexuality in civilizing our society.* As Dr. Prescott has concluded from his research, "Physical pleasure is not only moral, but morally necessary if we are to become moral persons and thus, a moral society."

Sexual Healing: What Can It Really Do?

Sam found that making love to his partner in the morning changed his mood for the whole day. He was more effective at the office because he could regulate tension better.

Marjorie had a migraine headache cured by a sensuous massage and slow, careful attention of her partner during sex.

Elise reported that her lover, with a chronic back problem, never suffered from this ailment again after a bonding experience they had during sex.

Paul, who had severe arthritis, said the pain was alleviated during arousal and orgasm because of his feeling that his body was light and floating, his limbs suspended in air.

Elliott had suffered with erectile problems in his first marriage. But when he began a relationship with his new lover, whom he eventually married, his dysfunction vanished, and with it the fatigue, lack of energy, and depression he'd lived with for the past five years.

How Does Our Sexuality Offer Healing Power?

- It restores our sense of harmony with self and the environment.

- Union with a partner assures us we are part of the wholeness of humanity.
- It allows us to create new life if we wish.
- It offers pain reduction via arousal and orgasm.
- It enhances self-esteem.
- Physical and emotional release reduce depression and anxiety.
- It is the trigger of hormonal influences throughout the body for lubrication and restoration.
- There is, quite possibly, an immune system response to sexual stimulation via neurotransmitters and hormones that have an affinity for immune cells.
- Brain cell stimulation results from bridging between left and right hemispheres during an ecstasy experience.

We Can Achieve a Balance Between Sex and Life

Sexuality offers a way of knowing, a sense of personal awareness that allows you to change the course of nature, if you want to. But you must not split off your powerful sexual feelings from the rest of life. Only by integrating the body and its passion with an intent to heal and grow, can you become a highly developed sexual being.

If you can extend sex out of the bedroom, into the world, you can do anything. Suppose you could get up after loving each other and do the taxes together! Now that would really be a bonding experience. Even if you fought about money, your argument would be charged with all that sexual tension that made things exciting between you earlier. Even if you got depressed about your financial picture, you would have that connection of being two in one that would carry you through.

You don't have to be part of a couple to make this happen. Your sexuality is like an invisible protective shield, a warm cloak that covers your insecurities, nourishes your good feelings about yourself, enhances your appearance, and gives flash to your personality. You can walk into a room and feel eyes on you because of this power you exude. You can give to others with it, charging them with your energy and enthusiasm. If you are a truly sexual being, the juices that flow from arousal to life will affect everyone and everything you touch.

Being sexual in daily life doesn't mean thinking about sex all the time; it does, however, mean putting yourself forward in a way you may not consciously know how to do. Listen to what different people have to say:

Drummond, a retired accountant who was widowed in his late seventies: "It finally occurred to me that I didn't have to miss sex so much. I could harness my sexuality and direct it to areas of my life that weren't sexual at all. I could use the feeling I got being around a beautiful young woman that would make the rest of my day, like I'd gotten a gift or as if I'd read a surprising thing in a book that really related to me."

Terry, a dancer in her twenties: "Sex is really my humanness—I can send it out whatever way I want."

Mark, a divorced carpenter in his late thirties: "I couldn't imagine myself not experiencing my true sexuality. I think the world would be gray without the true colors of my sex."

Rob, the sixty-two-year-old minister: "People who are sexual are blessed, they can remake themselves. They're a creative repository for all that sexual energy and they can take it in many directions, to build a new house, to attract a new person, to take an intellectual journey."

Suppose we think of sexuality as the life force itself, the spark within each of us that draws us into the fray, allows us to fight for what we stand for and take a lot of punches along the way. Some of us, those who have survived sexual abuse, in particular, come to this ability after a long, hard struggle. Having had their sexuality used for malicious purposes, they must heal themselves thoroughly before being able to use their gift again. People who form deep spiritual bonds with their beloved can't trust themselves to do it alone—they must feel connected to another before their true sexuality shines. Some unconventional lovers flaunt their sexuality because others haven't approved of it, and others shroud it over so that no one will suspect it's there. Those who throw themselves into the passionate life regardless of the risks involved appear to be the most comfortable using their sexuality outside the bedroom, but most of these are older individuals, having had years to hone their art and sharpen their desire.

You are sexy if you participate in this great game; and even if you have lost your way and have been suppressing your sexual nature for decades, there are many paths back. Good, clean, healthy sex pervades our lives, if we would just surrender ourselves to it as we do to a lover we trust and cherish. The abandon with which we can explore our sexuality will turn on the world.

Sexuality. Claim it for yourself. Make it a vibrant part of you. Live it every day.

Resource Guide

Recommended Reading

Ader, Robert and David Felton. *Psychoneuroimmunology,* 2nd ed. San Diego, CA: San Diego Press, 1990.

Anand, Margo. *The Art of Sexual Ecstasy.* New York: Tarcher/Perigee Books, 1989.

Barbach, Lonnie. *For Yourself: The Fulfillment of Female Sexuality.* Garden City: Doubleday, 1975.

Brecher, Edward M. and the Editors of Consumer Reports Books. *Love, Sex and Aging.* Mt. Vernon, NY: Consumer's Union, 1984.

Calderone, Mary and Eric W. Johnson. *The Family Book About Sexuality.* New York: Perennial Library, 1989, 1991.

Cassell, Carol. *Straight from the Heart.* New York: Fireside Books, 1987.

Cutler, Winnifred B. *Love Cycles: The Science of Intimacy.* New York: Villard Books, 1991.

Dennis, Wendy. *Hot and Bothered.* New York: Viking, 1992.

Ehrenreich, Barbara, Elizabeth Hess, and Gloria Jacobs. *Re-Making Love.* Garden City, NY: Anchor Press/Doubleday, 1986.

Feldenkrais, Moshe. *The Potent Self.* New York: HarperCollins, 1985.

Fisher, Helen E. *Anatomy of Love.* New York: W. W. Norton, 1992.

Francoeur, Robert. *Becoming a Sexual Person,* 2nd ed. New York: Macmillan, 1991.

285

Giddens, Anthony. *The Transformation of Intimacy*. Stanford, CA: Stanford University Press, 1992.

Greer, Germaine. *The Change*. New York: Alfred A. Knopf, 1991.

Hartman, William and Marilyn Fithian. *Any Man Can*. New York: St. Martins, 1984.

Heiman, Julia R. and Joseph Lopiccolo. *Becoming Orgasmic*. New York: Fireside Press, 1992.

Heyn, Dalma. *The Erotic Silence of the American Wife*. New York: Turtle Bay Books, 1992.

Highwater, Jamake. *Myth & Sexuality*. New York: Meridian/Penguin Books, 1991.

Hopson, Janet L. *Scent Signals*. New York: William A. Morrow, 1979.

Kinsey, Alfred C., et al. *Sexual Behavior in the Human Female*. Philadelphia and London: W. B. Saunders, 1953.

Kinsey, Alfred C., et al. *Sexual Behavior in the Human Male*. Philadelphia: W. B. Saunders, 1948.

Klein, Marty. *Ask Me Anything*. New York: Fireside, 1992.

Kroll, Ken and Erica Levy Kroll. *Enabling Romance: A Guide to Love, Sex and Relationships for the Disabled*. New York: Harmony Books, 1992.

McCain, Marian Van Eyk. *Transformation Through Menopause*. New York: Bergin & Garvey, 1991.

McIlvenna, Ted. *The Complete Guide to Safer Sex and Sex in the Age of AIDS*. San Francisco: Institute for the Advanced Study of Human Sexuality, 1987, 1992.

Margulis, Lynn and Dorion Sagan. *Mystery Dance*. New York: Summit Books, 1991.

Masters, William H., M.D., and Virginia E. Johnson. *Human Sexual Response*. Boston: Little, Brown, 1966.

May, Robert. *Sex and Fantasy*. New York: W. W. Norton, 1980.

Meshorer, Marc and Judith Meshorer. *Ultimate Pleasures: The Secrets of Easily Orgasmic Women*. New York: St. Martins, 1986.

Moyers, Bill. *Healing and the Mind*. New York: Doubleday, 1993.

Offit, Avodah K. *The Sexual Self*. New York: Ballantine Books, 1977.

Ornstein, Robert and David Sobel. *The Healing Brain*. New York: Touchstone Books, 1987.

Rosen, Raymond C. and Sandra R. Leiblum. *Erectile Disorders*. New York: The Guilford Press, 1992.

Sachs, Judith. *What Women Should Know About Menopause*. New York: Dell, 1991.

Sarrel, Phillip. *Sexual Turning Points*. New York: Macmillan, 1984.

Schover, L. and Jensen, S. *Sexuality and Chronic Illness*. New York: The Guilford Press, 1988.

Selby, John. *Peak Sexual Experience*. New York: Warner Books, 1992.

Sheehy, Gail. *The Silent Passage*. New York: G. Merritt, 1992.

Starr, Bernard D. and Marcella Bakur Weiner. *On Sex and Sexuality in the Mature Years*. New York: Stein & Day, 1981.

Stoppard, Miriam. *The Magic of Sex*. New York: Dorling Kindersley, 1992.

Thayer, Robert. *The Biopsychology of Mood and Arousal*. New York: Oxford University Press, 1989.

Timmerman, Joan H. *Sexuality and Spiritual Growth*. New York: The Crossroad Publishing Co., 1992.

Walz, Thomas H. and Nancee S. Blum. *Sexual Health In Later Life*. Lexington, MA: D. C. Heath, 1987.

Whipple, Beverly and Gina Ogden. *Safe Encounters*. New York: Pocket Books, 1990.

Woods, Nancy Fugate. *Human Sexuality in Health and Illness*, 3rd ed. St. Louis: C. V. Mosby, 1984.

Yaffe, Maurice and Elizabeth Fenwick. *Sexual Happiness for Men*. New York: Henry Holt, 1986, 1992.

Yaffe, Maurice and Elizabeth Fenwick. *Sexual Happiness for Women*. New York: Henry Holt, 1992.

Additional Resources

Information on Nonoxynol-15

Institute for Advanced Study of Human Sexuality
1523 Franklin St.
San Francisco, CA 94109

Information on Sex and Disability

It's Okay! a magazine on sexuality and disability, Linda Crabtree, Phoenix Counsel, Inc., 1 Springbank Drive, St. Catharines, Ontario, Canada, L2S 2K1, $23.95 a year.

Erotic Aids for Women

Eve's Garden
119 West 57th Street, Suite 420
New York, NY 10019
Catalog for $3.00.

Erotic Aids for Men and Women

Adam and Eve
One Apple Court
P.O. Box 800
Carrboro, NC 27510

Catalog arrives in brown paper wrapper.

Good Vibrations
938 Howard Street
San Francisco, CA 94103

Catalogue ($1) of aids, books and videos arrives in plain packaging.

Organizations Dedicated to Sex Education

National Society for the Scientific Study of Sex (SSSS)
P.O. Box 208
Mt. Vernon, IA 52314

Sex Education and Information Council of the US (SIECUS)
130 West 42nd Street, 25th floor
New York, NY 10036

American Association of Sex Educators, Counselors and Therapists (AASECT)
435 North Michigan Avenue, Suite 1717
Chicago, IL 60611

The Kinsey Institute for Research in Sex, Gender and Reproduction
University of Indiana
Morrison Hall 313
Bloomington, IN 47405-2501

$\mathcal{I}$ndex

CPSIA information can be obtained
at www.ICGtesting.com
Printed in the USA
BVHW042148140622
639826BV00002B/19

9 781504 028912